BRADY

PREHOSPITAL
EMERGENCY
PHARMACOLOGY

BRADY

PREHOSPITAL EMERGENCY PHARMACOLOGY

THIRD EDITION

BRYAN E. BLEDSOE, D.O.

Emergency Department Physician
Baylor Medical Center–Waxahachie
Waxahachie, Texas

GIDEON BOSKER, M.D., F.A.C.E.P.

Director, Continuing Education Programs
Member, Columbia Emergency Medicine Associates (CEMA)
Department of Emergency Medicine
Good Samaritan Hospital and Medical Center
Portland, Oregon

FRANK J. PAPA, D.O., Ph.D., F.A.C.E.P.

Associate Professor of Emergency Medicine and Medical Education
Department of Medical Education
Texas College of Osteopathic Medicine
University of North Texas
Fort Worth, Texas

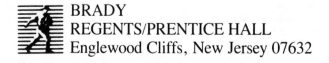
BRADY
REGENTS/PRENTICE HALL
Englewood Cliffs, New Jersey 07632

Library of Congress Cataloging-in-Publication Data

Bledsoe, Bryan E., 1955–
   Prehospital emergency pharmacology / Bryan E. Bledsoe, Gideon
Bosker, Frank J. Papa. — 3rd ed.
    p.   cm.
   Includes bibliographical references and index.
   ISBN 0–89303–949–7
   1. Medical emergencies. 2. Chemotherapy. 3. Drugs. I. Bosker,
Gideon. II. Papa, Frank J., 1949–   . III. Title.
   [DNLM: 1. Drug Therapy. 2. Emergencies. WB 105 B646p]
  RC86.7.B597 1992
  616.02'5—dc20
  DNLM/DLC
  for Library of Congress   91–35320
                                          CIP

Production editor: ADELE M. KUPCHIK   Prepress buyer: ILENE LEVY
Acquisitions editor: NATALIE ANDERSON   Manufacturing buyer: ED O'DOUGHERTY
Copy editor: ANDREA K. HAMMER   Editorial assistant: LOUISE FULLAM
Cover designer: LUNDGREN GRAPHICS

Notice: The author and the publisher of this book have taken care to make certain that the equipment, doses of drugs and schedules of treatment are correct and compatible with the standards generally accepted at the time of publication. Nevertheless, as new information becomes available, changes in treatment and in the use of equipment and drugs become necessary. The reader is advised to carefully consult the instruction and information material included in the package insert of each drug or therapeutic agent, piece of equipment or device before administration. This advice is especially important when using new or infrequently used drugs. No endorsement by the American Heart Association or any of its committees is stated or implied, nor is there any suggested warranty of performance during the American Heart Association Advanced Cardiac Life Support Course. Prehospital Care Providers are warned that use of any drugs or techniques must be authorized by their medical advisor, in accord with local laws and regulations. The publisher disclaims any liability, loss, injury, or damage incurred as a consequence, directly or indirectly, of the use and application of any of the contents of this book.

Printed in the United States of America

10 9 8 7 6 5 4 3 2

ISBN 0-89303-949-7

Prentice-Hall International (UK) Limited, *London*
Prentice-Hall of Australia Pty. Limited, *Sydney*
Prentice-Hall Canada Inc., *Toronto*
Prentice-Hall Hispanoamericana, S.A., *Mexico*
Prentice-Hall of India Private Limited, *New Delhi*
Prentice-Hall of Japan, Inc., *Tokyo*
Simon & Schuster Asia Pte. Ltd., *Singapore*
Editora Prentice-Hall do Brasil, Ltda., *Rio de Janeiro*

CONTENTS

6 DRUGS USED IN TREATMENT OF CARDIOVASCULAR EMERGENCIES 73

7 DRUGS USED IN TREATMENT OF RESPIRATORY EMERGENCIES

8 DRUGS USED IN TREATMENT OF METABOLIC-ENDOCRINE EMERGENCIES

PREFACE

Prehospital Emergency Pharmacology is a complete guide to the most common medications used in the prehospital phase of emergency medicine. The first edition was published in 1982 and has received widespread use in prehospital education programs. The text was designed with two purposes in mind. First, it is a complete pharmacology teaching text. Second, it is a handy reference to over 75 of the most common drugs and fluids used in prehospital care.

The third edition has been extensively updated to reflect current trends in prehospital care as well as American Heart Association Advanced Cardiac Life Support (ACLS) and Pediatric Advanced Life Support (PALS) standards. Many new medications have been added and several infrequently used medications have been deleted. American Heart Association ACLS treatment algorithms have been added to summarize management of cardiac emergencies. A complete pharmacologic glossary has also been added for rapid reference. The home medication reference guide has been completely revised and updated.

We hope that *Prehospital Emergency Pharmacology* will prove a valuable aid to both the practicing paramedic as well as the paramedic student.

AUTHORS' NOTE

ACKNOWLEDGMENTS

As *Prehospital Emergency Pharmacology* enters its third edition it is time again to acknowledge the many talented individuals who provided both support and assistance throughout all three editions of this text.

First, we would like thank Natalie Anderson, editor at Brady, for her assistance and support in this project. Adele Kupchik in College Book Editorial Production at Prentice Hall skillfully organized and supervised production of the third edition.

The authors would like to acknowledge the assistance provided by the reviewers of the third edition including Richard Cherry, M.Ed., EMT-P; Judith Creemens, R.N.; Robert S. Porter, M.A., EMT-P; and many others.

Paramedics from East Texas EMS served as models for the third edition photographs. Their assistance is deeply appreciated.

Finally, as with the two prior editions, the authors would like to thank Emma Bledsoe for her patience as well as her assistance in typing portions of the manuscript.

DISCLAIMER

The drugs presented in this text should only be administered under explicit medical control. EMS standards and levels of care vary significantly across this country and Canada. Paramedics should always refer to local standards and policies, as specified by the local medical director, regarding the administration of emergency medications and fluids. Some medications presented in this text may be appropriate for one system and inappropriate for another.

Every effort has been made to assure that information provided in this reference is accurate and complete at the time of publication. Dosages and routes are taken from the most recent American Heart Association *Advanced Cardiac Life Support (ACLS)* and *Pediatric Advanced Life Support (PALS)* standards, where applicable. Drugs not covered in ACLS and PALS standards are referenced to the *Physician's Desk Reference* or the American Medical Association's *Drug Evaluation*. Although the review process has been extensive, errors may be present. Also, the dosages, routes, and standards for emergency medications are revised periodically. **THEREFORE, IT IS THE RESPONSIBILITY OF EACH INDIVIDUAL TO BE FAMILIAR WITH THE EMERGENCY MEDICATIONS AND FLUIDS USED IN THEIR SYSTEM AS SPECIFIED BY THE SYSTEM MEDICAL DIRECTOR. THIS IS TO INCLUDE THE INDICATIONS, CONTRAINDICATIONS, DOSAGES, AND ROUTES.**

INFECTIOUS DISEASES

Infectious diseases such as Human Immunodeficiency Virus (HIV) infection, hepatitis B infection, and other illnesses pose an occupational risk for prehospital personnel. Because of this, all EMS personnel must adhere to the "Universal Precautions" for health care workers as published by the Centers for Disease Control. The use of Universal Precautions will serve to minimize the risk of infectious disease transmission. **ALWAYS USE "UNIVERSAL PRECAUTIONS" IN ANY PATIENT CARE SITUATION.**

1

GENERAL INFORMATION

INTRODUCTION

Drugs are chemical agents used in the diagnosis, treatment, or prevention of disease. The study of drugs and their actions on the body is called **pharmacology**. Scientists who study the effects of drugs on the body are called **pharmacologists**. It is through experimental pharmacology that medicine has made many of its most profound advances.

HISTORICAL CONSIDERATIONS

The use of drugs in the treatment of various medical disorders is as old as the practice of medicine itself. Written records of drug use date back to early Egyptian times. Hippocrates, generally considered the father of modern medicine, wrote extensively on the use of drugs, although he rarely used them in the care of his patients. Following the Renaissance, healers began to take a somewhat more scientific approach to disease, and found that certain drugs were useful in treating some disorders but not others. Drug therapy was largely empiric, and physicians were frequently unsure which body systems the drugs affected.

One common additive to medications was the Purple Foxglove plant. A common flowering plant, the Purple Foxglove was first described in A.D. 1250 by Welsh physicians. It was long thought to be a diuretic because

1

of its role in the treatment of dropsy, an old term used to describe the generalized body edema associated with congestive heart failure. In 1785, William Withering detailed the use of the Purple Foxglove plant in the treatment of dropsy and other disorders. Although he did not associate the improvement seen in the treatment of dropsy as being due to Foxglove's effect on the heart, he did note its effectiveness. He wrote, "It has a power over the motion of the heart to a degree yet unobserved in any other medicine." It was not until 1800 that the effect of Foxglove specifically on the heart was actually described and its suspected action as a diuretic was finally discarded.

Digitalis is the active agent in Foxglove. Digitalis tends to increase myocardial contractile force. It was this increase in cardiac performance with subsequently improved renal perfusion and filtration that caused a reduction in the body swelling, and not its diuretic effect as earlier thought. Even today digitalis is still one of the most commonly prescribed medications in the treatment of congestive heart failure and other cardiovascular disorders.

DRUG SOURCES

Drugs are derived from four primary sources. These include plant, animal, mineral, and synthetic. Emergency medications derived from **plant sources** include morphine sulfate and atropine sulfate among others. Morphine is made from parts of the opium plant, which is native to Turkey and other parts of the Middle East. In addition to morphine, heroin, codeine, and many other analgesic preparations are derived from the opium plant. Because of their psychotropic effects, these drugs are subject to abuse. They also can result in physical and psychological dependence.

Atropine sulfate, another drug derived from plant sources, is used in the treatment of slow heart rates. Atropine is derived from the plant *Atropa belladonna*.

Examples of drugs derived from **animal sources** include insulin and oxytocin. Both of these agents are endocrine hormones extracted from desiccated endocrine glands of mammals. Insulin is used in the treatment of diabetes mellitus, whereas oxytocin is used to induce labor and treat certain types of vaginal bleeding.

Two emergency medications come from **mineral (inorganic) sources**. They are sodium bicarbonate ($NaHCO_3$) and magnesium sulfate ($MgSO_4$). Sodium bicarbonate is sometimes used to treat severe metabolic acidosis. Magnesium sulfate is used in the treatment of eclampsia, a life-threatening seizure associated with pregnancy.

Most drugs on the market today are synthetically derived. The term **synthetic** means that they are made by people. Common examples of emergency drugs that are synthetically manufactured include lidocaine (Xylocaine®), bretylium tosylate (Bretylol®), diazepam (Valium®), and many others. Lidocaine and bretylium tosylate are antiarrhythmics. Valium® is used in the treatment of seizures and other neuropsychiatric disorders.

DRUG LEGISLATION

Before a drug can be marketed, it must undergo extensive testing. This testing generally involves two phases, animal studies and clinical patient studies. Only after these extensive tests, and with governmental approval, can drugs be placed on the market. Even after clinical usage, the efficacy of the drugs must be closely monitored. The Food and Drug Administration (FDA) is responsible for approval of drugs before they are made available to the general public.

The FDA enforces rigid standards imposed by various legislation. In 1906, Congress enacted the **Pure Food and Drug Act**. In addition to establishing the FDA, this act prohibited the sale of medicinal preparations that had little or no use, and restricted the sale of drugs with a potential for abuse. The Pure Food and Drug Act was not as all encompassing as its planners had envisioned it to be. For several years, stronger drug laws were debated both in Congress and state legislatures. Finally, in 1938, Congress enacted the **Federal Food, Drug and Cosmetic Act**. Among the more important features of this act was the truth-in-labeling clause. The act required that the names of all ingredients used in the preparation of the drug as well as directions for the drug's use must be indicated on the label. The label must also indicate whether or not the preparation contains habit-forming drugs and the percentage of those drugs present. Any drug bearing the official title U.S.P. (**United States Pharmacopeia**) or N.F. (**National Formulary**) must conform to certain rigid standards regarding purity, preparation, and dosage.

NARCOTICS

A problem almost as old as medicine itself is abuse and addiction to certain drugs. Narcotics are among the drugs most frequently abused. Recognizing the need to control the sale of narcotics, the federal government enacted the **Harrison Narcotic Act** in 1915. This act served to control the importation, manufacture, and sale of the opium plant and its derivatives. It also controlled the derivatives of the coca plant. The primary drug derived from the coca plant is cocaine. As a result of this act, these drugs, as well as other drugs added to the list later, could be obtained only with special prescriptions. Only physicians who qualified and attained a special narcotic license could prescribe this class of drugs.

In 1970, major revisions were made in the use and control of narcotics and other drugs. This law, the **Controlled Substance Act**, classifies the drugs used in medicine into five different schedules. A summary of the five schedules follow:

Schedule I. Drugs in this schedule have a high potential for abuse and no accepted medical usefulness. Drugs in this class include some derivatives of the opium plant (heroin), marijuana, synthetic opiates, and hallucinogenic drugs (LSD) among others. These drugs are used only in research.

Schedule II. Drugs in this schedule have a high potential for abuse, yet have accepted medical usefulness. Some opium preparations, synthetic narcotics and cocaine, as well as some amphetamines, are included in this group. Emergency drugs used by paramedics classified in Schedule II include morphine sulfate and meperidine (Demerol®).

Schedule III. Drugs having a lesser degree of abuse potential and accepted medical indications are classified as Schedule III. Drugs containing some narcotic ingredients are usually placed in this class. Codeine is a popular narcotic used to enhance the analgesic effects of other analgesic drugs. An example of this mixture is acetaminophen (Tylenol®) with codeine.

Schedule IV. Drugs having a low potential for abuse, but which may cause physical or psychological dependence, are placed in Schedule IV. Many of the depressants, stimulants, and sedatives are classified as Schedule IV. Valium® is an example of a Schedule IV drug.

Schedule V. Schedule V drugs are drugs that have low potential for abuse. Cough medications containing codeine as well as certain antidiarrheal agents that contain opiates are classified as Schedule V drugs.

The Controlled Substances Act mandates that prescriptions for Schedule II drugs cannot be refilled. Moreover, it requires that prescriptions for Schedule II drugs be filled within 72 hours. Prescriptions for drugs in this class cannot be called into the pharmacy over the telephone (except in special situations). Prescriptions for drugs in Schedules III and IV may be refilled up to 5 times within 6 months. Prescriptions for Schedule V drugs may be refilled at the discretion of the physician.

Responsibility for enforcing the Controlled Substances Act rests with the Drug Enforcement Administration (DEA). Only physicians approved by the DEA may write prescriptions for Scheduled drugs. The physician must indicate his or her DEA number on each when prescribing drugs in these classes.

DRUG NAMES

Drugs are identified by four different names: **chemical, generic, trade,** and **official**. The most elemental name is the chemical name. Because drugs are usually chemically complex in nature, so too are the chemical names. The **generic name**, usually an abbreviated version of the chemical name, is frequently used. Manufacturers of pharmaceuticals rarely refer to drugs by their generic name. Instead, they devise a name for a drug that is based on its chemical name or on the type of problem it is used to treat. This is referred to as the **trade name**. In recent years, controversy has developed regarding generic and nongeneric drugs. When writing a prescription, a physician can order the drug either by the trade name or the generic name. Until recently, the pharmacist had to fill the drug as written. Now, in many states, the pharmacist may substitute a less-expensive generic drug for the prescription. Generic drugs are, as a rule, not inferior in quality. They are usually cheaper because they are manufactured by lesser-known companies with minimal advertising and production costs. The fourth method of naming a drug is the **official name**. The official name is followed by the initials U.S.P. or N.F., which are official publications that list drugs conforming to standards set forth by the publication. The official name is usually the same as the generic name. An example of the four names of a specific drug is as follows:

Chemical Name ethyl 1-methyl-4-phenylisonipecotate hydrochloride
Generic Name meperidine hydrochloride
Trade Name Demerol® Hydrochloride
Official Name meperidine hydrochloride, U.S.P.

DRUG REFERENCES

Several publications provide valuable information concerning drugs. These include the following:

AMA Drug Evaluation. This manual, which is published by the American Medical Association, provides information on all drug groups and includes dosages, prescribing information, and usage.

Physicians' Desk Reference (PDR). The PDR is a valuable reference. It contains information concerning most of the drugs on the market today and a very useful product identification guide showing actual size and color pictures of commonly prescribed drugs. The PDR is published yearly by the Medical Economics Company.

Hospital Formulary. The Hospital Formulary is a loose-leaf book published by the American Society of Hospital Pharmacists. Its loose-leaf format allows it to be constantly updated, and is available in all hospital pharmacies and in most emergency departments.

Drug Inserts. The written literature packaged with most drugs are good sources of information. They can be collected and put into a notebook for personal use.

DRUG FORMS

Drugs come in many forms. Each drug has its advantages and disadvantages. For example, drugs taken by mouth tend to have a slow and unpredictable rate of absorption and thus a slower rate of onset. Drugs given intravenously, although rapidly acting, are much more difficult to administer. The following are some common drug preparations.

Liquids

Liquid drugs usually consist of a powder dissolved in a liquid. The drug is referred to as the **solute**. The liquid into which it is dissolved is called the **solvent**. In liquid drug preparations, the primary difference from one preparation to another is the solvent.

Solutions. Solutions are preparations where the drugs are dissolved in a solvent, usually water (for example, 5% dextrose in water).

Tinctures. Tinctures are drug preparations whereby the drug was extracted chemically with alcohol. They will usually contain some dilute alcohol (for example, tincture of iodine).

Suspensions. Suspensions are drugs that do not remain dissolved. After sitting for even short periods, these drugs will tend to separate. They must always be shaken well before use (for example, penicillin preparations).

Spirits. Spirit solutions contain volatile chemicals dissolved in alcohol (for example, spirit of ammonia).

Emulsions. Emulsions are preparations in which an oily substance is mixed with a solvent into which it does not dissolve. When mixed, it forms globules of fat floating in the solvent. This is similar to what occurs in oil and vinegar salad dressing.

Elixirs. Elixirs are preparations that contain the drug in an alcohol solvent. Flavoring, usually cherry, is added to improve the taste (for example, Tylenol Elixer).

Syrups. Often drugs are suspended in sugar and water to improve the taste. These are referred to as syrups (for example, cough syrup).

Liquid drugs administered into the body through either intramuscular, subcutaneous, or intravenous routes are called **parenteral** drugs. Most drugs used in emergency medicine are parenteral. Because they are introduced into the body, they must be sterile. They are packaged in several types of containers. Sterile parenteral containers designed to carry a single patient dose are called **ampules** (see Figure 1–1). Generally, ampules are broken, and the drug is drawn into a syringe for administration.

In emergency medicine, most drugs given parenterally are in **prefilled** syringes (see Figure 1–2). These preparations save time by avoiding the problems inherent to ampules.

Wyeth manufactures a type of syringe called **Tubex®** (see Figure 1–3). This syringe is designed for a disposal cartridge containing the desired drug and is reusable. Several of the medications used in the emergency department and the field, including morphine and meperidine, are frequently carried in Tubex form.

Another type of container for parenteral drugs are **vials** (see Figures 1–4 and 1–5). Vials may contain a single dose or multiple dosages. Many drugs used in emergency medicine are supplied in vials.

Solid Drugs

Solid drugs are usually administered orally, although many can be administered rectally. They include the following:

Pills. Pills are drugs that are shaped into a form that makes them easy to swallow.

Powders. Powders are drugs in powdered form. They are not as popular as pills, yet some are still in use (for example, B.C. Powder®).

Capsules. Capsules consist of gelatin containers into which a powder is placed. The gelatin dissolves liberating the powder (for example, Dalmane® capsules) into the gastrointestinal tract.

Tablets. Tablets are similar to pills. They are composed of a powder that has been compressed into an easily swallowed form and are often covered with a sugar coating to improve taste.

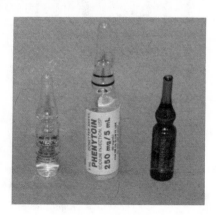

Figure 1–1 Examples of medications supplied in ampules.

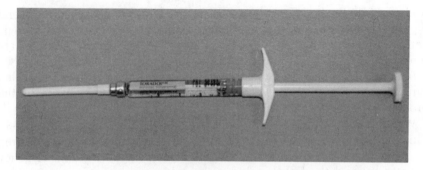

Figure 1–2 Example of a prefilled syringe.

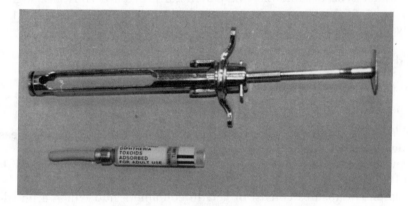

Figure 1–3 Tubex medication system.

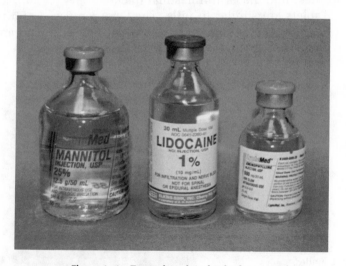

Figure 1–4 Examples of multiple dosage vials.

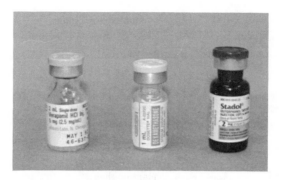

Figure 1–5   Examples of single dose vials.

Suppositories. Suppositories are mixed into a base that is solid at room temperature (approximately 70°F). When placed into the body, either rectally or vaginally, they dissolve and are then absorbed into the surrounding tissue.

COMMON PHARMACOLOGICAL TERMINOLOGY AND ABBREVIATIONS

It is common to use abbreviations in pharmacology. This serves to expedite paper work and promote efficiency. The abbreviations used in pharmacology are fairly standard. It is important to be familiar with these abbreviations and with some of the common terminology applicable to the field of emergency pharmacology (see Table 1–1).

Important Pharmacological Terminology

Antagonism. Antagonism signifies the opposition between two or more medications (for example, between Narcan® and morphine).

Bolus. A bolus is a single, oftentimes large dose of medication (for example, lidocaine bolus, which is often followed by a lidocaine infusion).

Contraindications. Contraindications are the medical or physiological conditions present in a patient that would make it harmful to administer a medication of otherwise known therapeutic value.

Cumulative Action. A cumulative action occurs when a drug is administered in several doses, causing an increased effect. This is usually due to a quantitative buildup of the drug in the blood.

Depressant. A depressant is a medication that decreases or lessens a body function or activity.

Habituation. Habituation is the physical or psychological dependence on a drug.

TABLE 1–1   **Common Abbreviations**

Abbreviation	Meaning
$\bar{a}$	*ante* (before)
a.c.	*ante cibos* (before meals)
ACh	acetylcholine
ACLS	advanced cardiac life support
admin.	administer
α	alpha
ALS	advanced life support
amp.	ampule
APAP	acetaminophen
ASA	aspirin
β	beta
bid	*bis in die* (twice a day)
$\bar{c}$	*cum* (with)
Ca^{++}	calcium ion
$CaCl_2$	calcium chloride
caps	capsules
cc	cubic centimeter
CC	chief complaint
CHF	congestive heart failure
Cl^-	chloride ion
cm	centimeter
cm^3	cubic centimeter
c/o	complains of
CO	carbon monoxide
CO_2	carbon dioxide
COPD	chronic obstructive pulmonary disease
CSM	carotid sinus massage
CVA	cerebrovascular accident
°	degree
°C	degrees Celsius
D/C	discontinue
↓	decrease
D_5W	5% dextrose in water
$D_{10}W$	10% dextrose in water
$D_{50}W$	50% dextrose in water
dig	digitalis
Dx	diagnosis
ECG	electrocardiogram
EKG	electrocardiogram
elix	elixir
EOA	esophageal obturator airway
=	equal to
et	and
ET	endotracheal
ETOH	alcohol (ethyl)
°F	degrees Fahrenheit
♀	female
g	gram
gr	grain

TABLE 1–1   **Common Abbreviations (continued)**

Abbreviation	Meaning
>	greater than
gtt	*gutta* (drop)
gtts	*guttae* (drops)
HHN	hand-held nebulizer
hs	*hora somni* (at bedtime)
↑	increase
IC	intracardiac
IM	intramuscular
IO	intraosseous
IV	intravenous
IVP	intravenous push
IVPB	intravenous piggyback
K^+	potassium
kg	kilogram
KO	keep open
KVO	keep vein open
l	liter
lb	pound
<	less than
LR	lactated Ringer's
♂	male
MAX	maximum
MDI	metered dose inhaler
μ	micro
μgtt	microdrop
μg	microgram
mcg	microgram
μm	micrometer
mEq	milliequivalent
mg	milligram
min	minute
ml	milliliter
mm	millimeter
MS	morphine sulfate
MSO_4	morphine sulfate
N_2O	nitrous oxide
Na^+	sodium ion
$NaHCO_3$	sodium bicarbonate
nitro	nitroglycerin
NKA	no known allergies
NKDA	no known drug allergies
NTG	nitroglycerin
ø	null or none
O_2	oxygen
OD	overdose
OPP	organophosphate poisoning
OD	*oculus dexter* (right eye)
OS	*oculus sinister* (left eye)
OU	*oculus utro* (both eyes)

TABLE 1–1   **Common Abbreviations (continued)**

Abbreviation	Meaning
oz	ounce
p̄	*post* (after)
pc	*post cibos* (after eating)
PAC	premature atrial contraction
PAT	paroxysmal atrial tachycardia
pedi	pediatric
PJC	premature junctional contraction
po	*per os* (by mouth)
pr	*per rectus* (by rectum)
prn	*pro re nata* (when necessary)
PSVT	paroxysmal supraventricular tachycardia
q̄	*quisque* (every)
qd	*quisque die* (every day)
qh	*quisque hora* (every hour)
qid	*quater in die* (four times a day)
qod	every other day
qt	quart
®	registered trademark
RL	Ringer's lactate
Rx	treatment
s̄	*sine* (without)
SC	subcutaneous
SL	sublingual
sol	solution
SQ	subcutaneous
stat	*statim* (now or immediately)
SVN	small volume nebulizer
tid	*ter in die* (three times a day)
TKO	to keep open
u	unit
ut dict	*ut dictum* (as directed)
y/o	year old

Hypersensitivity. Hypersensitivity is a reaction to a substance that is normally more profound than seen in the normal population (for example, allergic reaction to penicillin).

Idiosyncrasy. An idiosyncrasy is an individual reaction to a drug that is unusually different from that seen in the rest of the population.

Indication. An indication refers to the medical condition(s) in which the drug has proven to be of therapeutic value.

Potentiation. Potentiation is the enhancement of one drug's effects by another (that is, barbiturates and alcohol).

Refractory. Patients who do not respond to a drug are said to be refractory to the drug (for example, a patient with premature ventricular contractions who does not respond to lidocaine).

Side Effects. Side effects are the unavoidable, undesired effects frequently seen even in therapeutic drug dosages.

Stimulant. A stimulant is a drug that enhances or increases a bodily function (for example, caffeine in coffee).

Synergism. Synergism is the combined action of two drugs. The action is much stronger than the effects of either drug administered separately.

Therapeutic Action. A therapeutic action is the desired, intended action of a drug given in the appropriate medical condition.

Tolerance. When patients are receiving drugs on a long-term basis, they may require larger and larger dosages of the drug to achieve a therapeutic effect. This increased requirement is termed tolerance.

Untoward Effect. An untoward effect is a side effect that proves harmful to the patient.

SUMMARY

Drugs are necessary for successful emergency care. It is important to be familiar with the commonly used emergency medications and with the terminology and abbreviations used in medicine so that communication with other medical personnel will be efficient and professional. Overall, it is essential to appreciate the inherent danger of any and all drugs, and to use them properly. The rule to remember is: When in doubt, *do no harm.*

2

PHARMACODYNAMICS AND PHARMACOKINETICS

INTRODUCTION

To exert its desired biochemical and physiological effects on the body, a drug must reach its targeted tissues in a suitable form and in a sufficient concentration. The study of how drugs enter the body, reach their site of action, and are eventually eliminated is termed **pharmacokinetics**. Once drugs reach their targeted tissues they begin a chain of biochemical events that ultimately lead to the physiological changes desired. These biochemical and physiological events are called the drug's **mechanism of action**. The study of drug actions is termed **pharmacodynamics**. This chapter addresses the fundamentals of both pharmacokinetics and pharmacodynamics as they apply to prehospital emergency care.

PHARMACOKINETICS

To produce its desired effects, a drug must be present in the appropriate concentration at its various sites of action. Lidocaine, a drug commonly used in the treatment of life-threatening ventricular dysrhythmias, must reach its target—cardiac tissue—rapidly and in a sufficient concentration to suppress the dysrhythmia. Several factors influence the concentration of a drug at its site of action. These factors include **absorption** of the drug into the circulatory system; **distribution** of the drug throughout the body;

biotransformation of the drug into its active form, if required; and finally, **elimination** of the drug from the body. It is important to point out that all of these factors do not play a role in every medication used in pre-hospital care. A fundamental understanding of each of these factors is essential.

Drug Absorption

Most medications used in general medical care are designed to be given by mouth. Once in the digestive system these medications are absorbed into the circulation and eventually transported to their various sites of actions. Administration of drugs by this route is generally safer, more convenient, and usually satisfactory in most instances. Absorption of a drug by the oral route is also much slower, however, and the eventual concentration of the drug in the circulation is often quite unpredictable. In an emergency situation, drugs must rapidly reach their site of action so they may quickly initiate the desired effects. Therefore, the administration of medications by the oral route is generally not acceptable in the emergency setting.

Medications used in prehospital care are generally given by either the intravenous, intramuscular, or subcutaneous routes (see Figure 2–1). When a drug is administered into either a muscle or the subcutaneous tissue it must be absorbed, through the walls of the capillaries, into the circulation, so that it can be subsequently transported to its sites of action. Some medications are placed near their site of action and have very few systemic effects. Examples of these drugs include the bronchodilators,

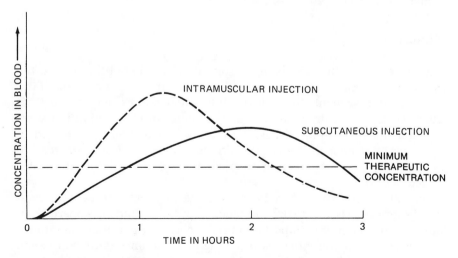

Figure 2–1 Comparison of drug levels following intramuscular and subcutaneous injections of the same drug.

which are administered by inhalation. Once inhaled, these medications immediately reach their target tissue (the lungs) and cause the desired effect.

Several factors may affect the rate at which the medication is absorbed. Factors that may *delay* absorption from parenteral sites include shock, acidosis, and peripheral vasoconstriction secondary to such things as hypothermia. Factors such as peripheral vasodilation, which can occur in hyperthermia and fever, may *increase* the rate of drug absorption. Muscles, as a rule, are more richly supplied with blood vessels than is subcutaneous tissue. Therefore, one would expect a drug to be absorbed more rapidly from muscle than from subcutaneous tissue. Knowledge of the various rates of drug absorption from each of the various routes is essential. Epinephrine 1:1000, a drug commonly used in the management of the acute stage of asthma, is generally given by the subcutaneous route. The reasons for choosing this site are many. First, epinephrine 1:1000 is a potent and concentrated drug. Rapid absorption of a large quantity of this drug into the circulation would certainly accentuate epinephrine's side effects such as tachycardia, trembling, and elevated blood pressure. Second, the therapeutic effects of epinephrine are fairly brief. The slower absorption obtained with subcutaneous injection allows prolonged release of the drug into the circulation, thus maintaining bronchodilation for a longer period (see Table 2–1).

Drug absorption may be minimized by injecting the medication directly into the circulatory system by the intravenous route. The desired effects are seen much sooner, and the eventual blood levels of the drug are much more predictable. Because of this, most critical-care medications are given intravenously (see Figure 2–2).

Distribution

Once a drug is in the circulatory system it is distributed throughout the various body tissues. Most drugs tend to pass fairly easily from the intravascular compartment, through the interstitial spaces, and on to their target tissue. These drugs tend to have a rapid onset of action but short duration of effect. Some drugs, conversely, are immediately bound to serum proteins after they enter the circulation. These drugs thus tend to have a delayed onset of action and remain in the circulation for a prolonged period.

Generally, drugs will tend to concentrate in those tissues with good blood supplies. Tissues with good blood supplies include the heart, liver, kidneys, and brain. It is important to remember that in critical situations, such as shock, the only tissues receiving blood to any significant extent are the heart and brain. Delivery of drugs to the brain is limited by what

TABLE 2–1   Comparison of Rates of Drug Absorption of Various Routes of Administration

Route	Rate of Absorption
Oral	Slow
Subcutaneous	Slow
Intramuscular	Moderate
Intravenous	Very rapid
Sublingual	Rapid
Transtracheal	Rapid
Inhalation	Rapid
Intracardiac	Immediate

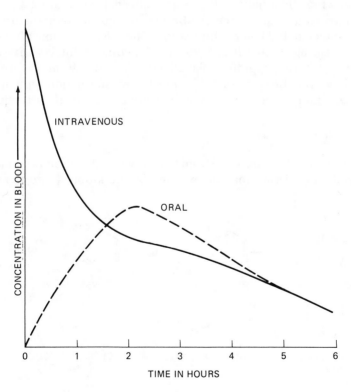

Figure 2–2 Comparison of drug levels following intravenous and oral administration of the same drug.

is called the **blood brain barrier**, which only allows entry of certain drugs and is considered a protective mechanism of the brain. Drugs that are protein bound or in an ionized form are weak penetrators of the blood brain barrier.

Biotransformation

Many drugs used in medicine are inactive when administered. Once they have been absorbed, they are then converted to an active form, either in the blood or by the target tissue. The process of changing a drug to another form, either active or inactive, is referred to as **biotransformation**. Biotransformation of drugs results in chemical variations of the drugs, which are called **metabolites**.

Several drugs used in prehospital care must be converted into an active form before they can exert their desired effects. Diazepam (Valium®), a drug used in the treatment of seizures, is relatively inactive as administered. Once in the body it is converted to its active metabolite, desmethyldiazepam, which then induces the desired effects (see Figure 2–3).

Some medications are active as administered but are biotransformed to an inactive metabolite before elimination. The liver is the most important organ for clearing metabolites. For example, epinephrine is active as administered. It is very rapidly metabolized to inactive forms before elimination, however. Because of this rapid biotransformation, epinephrine must be readministered approximately every 5 minutes if still required.

Elimination

Drugs are eventually eliminated from the body in either their original form or as metabolites. Drugs may be excreted by the kidneys into the urine,

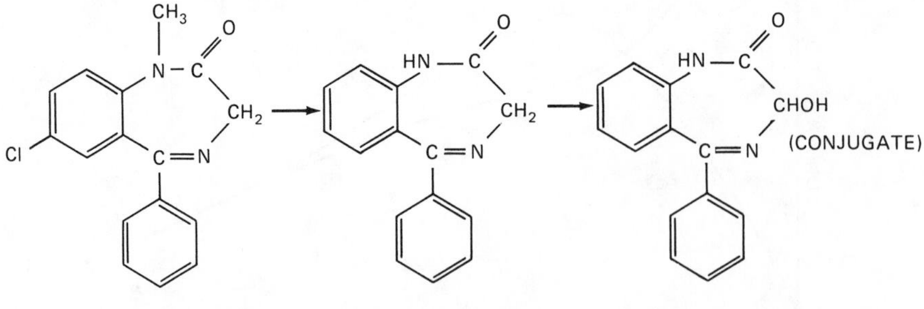

DIAZEPAM (VALIUM) — DESMETHYLDIAZEPAM — GLUCOURONIC ACID CONJUGATE

MINIMALLY ACTIVE — ***ACTIVE*** — ***INACTIVE***

Figure 2–3 Metabolites of diazepam.

by the liver into the bile, by the intestines into the feces, or by the lungs with the expired air. The rate of elimination varies with the medication and the state of the body. During shock states the kidneys are poorly perfused. Drugs that are primarily eliminated by the kidneys will then remain present in the body for longer periods. The slower the rate of elimination, the longer the drug stays in the body.

PHARMACODYNAMICS

Once a drug has arrived at the target tissue it must induce the desired biochemical or physiological response. Most drugs must bind to **drug receptors** to cause their desired response. Drug receptors are generally proteins present on the surface of the cell membrane. Drug receptors are often compared with "locks," whereas drugs are the "keys" that fit these locks. Once the drug is bound to the receptor (that is, the "key" is inserted in the "lock"), biochemical actions begin that ultimately lead to the desired response. Drugs that bind to a receptor and cause a response are referred to as **agonists**. Certain drugs, however, may bind to a receptor and not cause a response. Because of their presence on the receptor, they keep other drugs from binding. Drugs such as these are referred to as **antagonists**. Classic illustrations of this principle are the drugs epinephrine and propranolol (Inderal®). Epinephrine, once administered, is transported to its various target tissues—namely, the heart, the lungs, and the peripheral blood vessels. Once at these target tissues it finds and binds to its receptors, which are called **beta receptors**. If the drug is able to bind to these beta receptors then the desired physiological response will be seen. Several drugs themselves are inactive but can bind to beta receptors in much the same manner as epinephrine. These drugs are referred to as **beta blockers**, and the prototype drug of this group is propranolol. If a beta blocker has already bound to the receptor, then epinephrine cannot bind, and the desired effect is effectively blocked (see Figures 2–4 and 2–5). A more detailed discussion of beta receptors and beta blockers can be found in Chapter 6.

Once again, for a medication to be effective it must reach a certain concentration at the target tissue. The minimal concentration of a drug necessary to cause the desired response is referred to as the **therapeutic threshold** or **minimum effective concentration**. A concentration below this therapeutic threshold will not induce a clinical response. There is also a point at which the drug concentration can get high enough to be toxic or even fatal. The general goal of drug therapy is to give the minimum concentration of a drug necessary to obtain the desired response (see Figure 2–6).

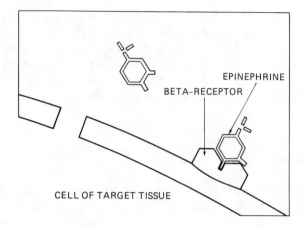

Figure 2–4   Epinephrine interacting with β receptor.

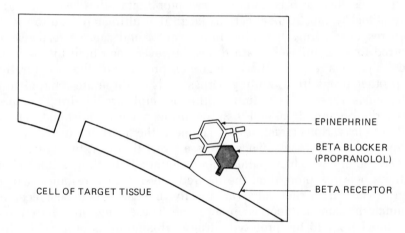

Figure 2–5   β Receptor blocked by propranolol.

The difference between the minimum effective concentration and the toxic level varies significantly from drug to drug. The difference between these two concentrations is referred to as the **therapeutic index** and is usually obtained in the laboratory. Certain drugs, such as digitalis, have very little difference between the effective dose and the toxic dose. Such drugs are said to have a low therapeutic index. Drugs such as naloxone (Narcan®), the narcotic antagonist, have a significant margin between the effective dose and the toxic dose, and are said to have a high therapeutic index. Prehospital care providers should be familiar with the therapeutic indices of the medications they use.

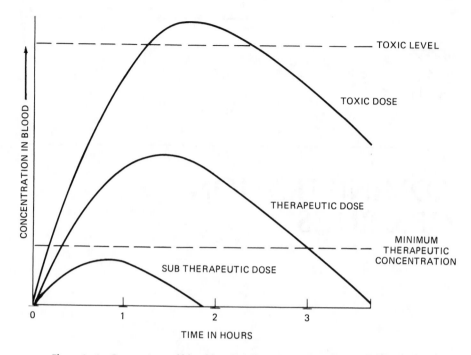

Figure 2–6   Comparison of blood levels following subtherapeutic, therapeutic, and toxic doses of the same drug.

SUMMARY

A basic understanding of pharmacokinetics and pharmacodynamics is essential for prehospital personnel to anticipate the desired therapeutic effects as well as any possible side effects of the medications they administer. Such factors as rate of absorption, elimination, minimum therapeutic concentration, and toxic levels should be considered in all drugs.

3

ADMINISTRATION OF DRUGS

INTRODUCTION

In the field of emergency medicine, medications must be administered promptly, in the correct dose, and by the correct route. Many drugs, although having therapeutic value when given by the appropriate route, can be fatal when given by another. Isoproterenol, for example, is a potent drug used to treat severe bradycardias. It is designed to be given by slow, intravenous infusion. If given in an intravenous bolus, however, it may be fatal. This admonition applies to most medications used in emergency medicine.

This chapter investigates the common routes and techniques for administration of medications used in emergency medical practice.

GENERAL ADMINISTRATION ROUTES

The two primary channels for getting medications into the body are through the alimentary canal (or digestive tract) and by parenteral routes. In acute care medicine, administration is almost always parenteral because the onset of action is much quicker and, usually, more predictable.

The following is a comparison of the relative advantages and disadvantages of alimentary versus parenteral administration.

Alimentary Tract

Advantages

1. Simple
2. Safe
3. Generally less expensive
4. Low potential for infection

Disadvantages

1. Slow rate of onset
2. Cannot be given to unconscious or nauseated patients
3. The absorbed dosage may vary significantly because of actions of digestive enzymes and the condition of the intestinal tract.

Parenteral

Advantages

1. Rapid onset
2. Can be given to unconscious and nauseated patients
3. Absorbed dosage, and action is more predictable.

Disadvantages

1. Administration is often difficult and painful
2. Usually more expensive
3. Side effects usually more severe.
4. Potential for infection

Alimentary Tract Routes

The common routes of alimentary tract administration used in general medical practice are as follows:

Oral. The best, and most convenient, way of administering drugs is by mouth. Most drugs in medicine are available in oral preparations. The effects of oral administration are often not seen until 30 to 45 minutes after administration.

Sublingual. Some drugs can be administered sublingually (that is, under the tongue). When administered in this fashion, the drug is placed under the tongue where it quickly dissolves. The drug is then absorbed into the vast capillary network present in the mucous membranes. Nitroglycerin, a drug frequently used in the management of angina pectoris, is administered by this route.

Rectal. Rectal administration may have both local and systemic effects. It may be necessary to administer some medications rectally, especially if the patient is nauseated. The rectal route is frequently used in infants and children who may not be able to swallow oral medications. Absorption of rectally administered drugs is generally somewhat slower than by the oral route.

Parenteral Routes

Any method of administration that does not involve passage through the digestive tract is termed parenteral. Parenteral routes include the following:

Intradermal. Drugs can be injected into the dermal layer of the skin. The amount of medication that can be given via this route is limited and systemic absorption (into the blood stream) is very slow. Generally, this route is reserved for diagnostic skin tests, like allergy testing.

Subcutaneous. With subcutaneous administration, medications are injected into fatty, subcutaneous tissue under the skin and overlying muscle. The rate of absorption is slower than that seen with intramuscular and intravenous administration. Epinephrine 1:1000, which is used in the treatment of acute asthma and other respiratory emergencies, is almost always administered subcutaneously. A maximum of 2 milliliters of a drug can be given subcutaneously.

Intramuscular. The most commonly used route of parenteral medication administration is the intramuscular route. The drug is injected into muscle tissue from which it is absorbed into the bloodstream. This method of administration has a predictable rate of absorption but is considerably slower than intravenous administration.

Intravenous. Most medications used in emergency medicine are designed to be administered intravenously. These can be in the form of an intravenous (IV) bolus or as a slow IV infusion, sometimes referred to as a piggyback infusion. The rate of absorption is rapid and predictable. Of all the routes frequently employed, however, IV administration of drugs has the most potential for causing adverse reactions.

Endotracheal. When an IV line cannot be started, it is sometimes possible to administer emergency medications down an endotracheal tube, which permits absorption into the capillaries of the lungs. It has been shown that this route has a rate of absorption as fast as the IV route. Drugs that can be administered endotracheally include epinephrine, lidocaine, naloxone, and atropine.

Sublingual Injection. In the rare instance where neither an IV line can be started nor an endotracheal tube inserted, certain drugs can be injected into the vast capillary network immediately under the tongue. Lidocaine is the agent most frequently given by this route.

Intracardiac. Injection of a medication directly into the ventricle of the heart is referred to as intracardiac administration. Because of the many complications associated with this procedure, it is reserved exclusively for life-threatening situations, such as cardiac arrest, when an IV line cannot be established nor an endotracheal tube placed.

Intraosseous. When an IV line cannot be started in children under 2 years of age, many emergency medications can be administered intraosseously. A needle can be placed in the anterior aspect of the proximal tibia through which medications and fluids can be administered. The onset of action is similar to IV administration.

Inhalational. Medications can be administered directly into the respiratory tree in cases of respiratory distress resulting from reversible airway disease including asthma and certain types of chronic obstructive pulmonary disease. These medications are usually nebulized into a water vapor and breathed with normal respiration.

MEDICATION ROUTES USED IN EMERGENCY MEDICINE

Emergency medications, with few exceptions, are administered parenterally by either the subcutaneous, intramuscular, intravenous, transtracheal, or intracardiac routes. Always use universal precautions in patient care, particularly with drug administration. The following section outlines the procedure for administration by each of these routes:

SUBCUTANEOUS INJECTION

Epinephrine 1:1000 is the emergency drug most frequently given subcutaneously. The procedure is as follows:

1. Receive order.
2. Confirm the order and write it down.
3. Prepare the necessary equipment and don gloves:
   - 1-cc syringe
   - Needle (preferably ⅝ inch in length, 25 gauge)
   - Alcohol preparation or other antibacterial swab
   - 4 × 4 gauze pad
   - Medication
4. Explain to the patient what you are going to do. Be sure to warn him or her of any complications that might result from the administration.
5. Reconfirm that the patient is not allergic to the medication you are going to administer.

6. Examine the ampule of medication, reconfirming that it is correct. Hold it up to the light and inspect for discoloration or particles in the solution. Do not administer if discolored or if particles are present.
7. "Shake down" the ampule. This will force the liquid to the lower portion of the ampule so that it can be broken without spillage of the drug.
8. Break the ampule using a 4 × 4 gauze pad to prevent injury.
9. Draw the medication into the syringe. Invert the syringe and expel any air present.
10. Choose a suitable site. The easiest and most accessible site is the subcutaneous tissue over the deltoid muscle in the arm (see Figure 3–1).
11. Insert the needle into the tissue at a 45° angle. (see Figure 3–2).

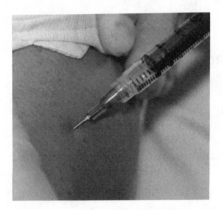

Figure 3–1 The needle should enter the skin at a 45° angle.

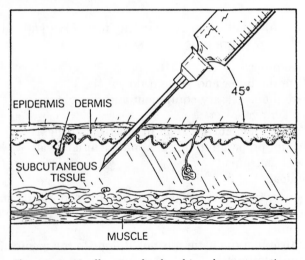

Figure 3–2 Needle properly placed in subcutaneous tissue.

12. Aspirate the syringe to assure that you are not in a blood vessel. If you get any blood return, you should withdraw the needle and reattempt administration at another site.
13. Inject the medication slowly.
14. Remove the syringe. Do not recap the needle.
15. Apply pressure to the site.
16. Cover with an adhesive strip.
17. Confirm administration of the medication.
18. Closely monitor the patient for the desired therapeutic effect and possible side effects.

Intramuscular Injection

Intramuscular injection is useful when rapid drug action is not required. The most common muscles into which drugs are administered are the deltoid and the gluteal. A maximum of 1 milliliter of medication can be given into the deltoid, whereas 10 milliliters can be given into the gluteal.

Medications can be given intramuscularly using the standard syringe, the Tubex® system, or prefilled syringes. The procedure for intramuscular medication administration is as follows:

1. Receive order.
2. Confirm the order and write it down.
3. Prepare the necessary equipment and don gloves:
   • Syringe of sufficient size to contain the medication
   • Needle (preferably ¾ to 1 inch in length, 21 to 25 gauge)
   • Alcohol preparation or other antibacterial swab
   • 4 × 4 gauze pad
   • Medication
4. Explain to the patient what you are going to do. Be sure to warn him or her of any complications that might result from the administration.
5. Reconfirm that the patient is not allergic to the medication you are going to administer.
6. Examine the ampule of medication, reconfirming that it is correct. Hold it up to the light and inspect for discoloration or particles in the solution. If the medication is discolored do not administer it.
7. "Shake down" the ampule. This will force the liquid to the lower portion of the ampule so that it can be broken without spillage of the drug.
8. Break the ampule using a 4 × 4 gauze pad to prevent injury.
9. Draw the medication into the syringe. Invert the syringe and expel any air present.

10. Choose a suitable site. The easiest and most accessible site is the deltoid muscle in the arm (see Figure 3–3).
11. Insert the needle into the tissue at a 90° angle (see Figure 3–4).
12. Aspirate the syringe to assure that you are not in a blood vessel. If you get any blood return, you should withdraw the needle and reattempt administration at another site.
13. Inject the medication slowly.
14. Remove the syringe. Do not recap the needle.
15. Apply pressure to the site.
16. Cover with an adhesive strip.
17. Confirm administration of the medication.
18. Closely monitor the patient for the desired therapeutic effect and possible undesired side effects.

It is important to note that, as a rule, patients presenting with a chief complaint of chest pain should not receive medications by the intramuscular route. Intramuscular injection of medication may cause an elevation of certain muscle enzymes that routinely circulate in the blood. In the emergency department these enzymes are frequently measured to determine whether the chest pain is of myocardial origin. An intramuscular injection in the prehospital phase of emergency medical care can cause a false elevation of these enzymes, which can subsequently confuse the emergency department physicians as he or she attempts to determine the etiology of the chest pain. There may be occasions, however, when the medical control physician may permit intramuscular injections when no other immediate route is available, and administration of the medication is essential.

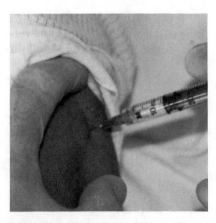

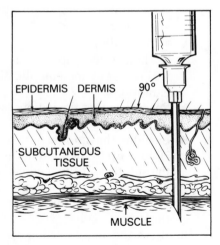

EPIDERMIS DERMIS   90°

SUBCUTANEOUS
    TISSUE

MUSCLE

Figure 3–3 The needle should enter the skin at a 90° angle.

Figure 3–4 Needle properly placed in muscle tissue.

Intravenous Administration

As mentioned previously, there, are two distinct methods of IV medication administration: (1) the IV bolus and (2) slow IV infusion (sometimes called "piggyback").

Emergency medications administered by the IV bolus technique are usually administered with prefilled syringes. Many medications, however, are still available only in ampule or vial form.

In all but a few cases, it is essential that an IV be established before administering medications intravenously. This makes the repeated administration of intravenous medications less traumatic.

IV Bolus

1. Receive the order.
2. Confirm the order and write it down.
3. Prepare the necessary equipment and don gloves:
   - Syringe of sufficient size to contain the medication
   - Needle (preferably 1 inch long, 18 gauge)
   - Alcohol preparation or other antibacterial swab
   - Adhesive bandage strip
   - Medication
4. Explain to the patient what you are going to do. Be sure to warn him or her of any complications that might arise as a result of the administration.
5. Reconfirm that the patient is not allergic to the medication that you are going to administer.
6. Examine the ampule of medication, reconfirming that it is correct. Hold it up to light and inspect for discoloration or particles in the solution. Do not administer the medication if discolored or if particles are present.
7. "Shake down" the ampule. This will force the liquid to the lower portion of the ampule so that it can be broken without spillage of the drug.
8. Break the ampule using a 4 × 4 gauze pad to prevent injury.
9. Draw the medication into the syringe. Invert the syringe and expel any air.
10. Locate the medication port on the IV administration set, and cleanse it with antibacterial solution.
11. Insert the needle into the medication port.
12. Pinch the IV line off above the medication port (see Figure 3–5).
13. Administer the medication in a slow, deliberate fashion.
14. Remove the needle and wipe the medication port with antibacterial solution.
15. Release the pinched line.

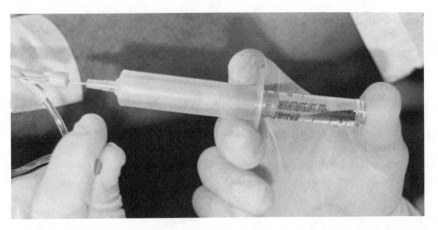

Figure 3–5 Pinch the IV line above the medication port before administering the medication.

16. Confirm administration of the medication.
17. Closely monitor the patient for the desired therapeutic effects as well as any undesired side effects.

IV Piggyback Administration

1. Receive the order.
2. Confirm the order and write it down.
3. Prepare the necessary equipment and don gloves:
   - Medication
   - Syringe to transfer the medication from the ampule to the dilutent
   - Alcohol prep or other antibacterial scrub
   - Two 18-gauge, 1-inch needles
   - Label for the bag
4. Explain to the patient what you are going to do. Be sure to warn him or her of any complications that might arise as a result of the administration.
5. Reconfirm that the patient is not allergic to the medication that you are going to administer.
6. Examine the ampule of medication, reconfirming that it is correct. Hold it up to light and inspect for discoloration or particles in the solution. Do not administer if discolored or if particles are present.
7. "Shake down" the ampule. This will force the liquid to the lower portion of the ampule so that it can be broken without spillage of the medication.
8. Break the ampule using a 4 × 4 gauze pad to prevent injury.
9. Draw the medication into the syringe using aseptic technique. Invert and expel any air.

10. Cleanse the medication port on the IV bag into which the medication will be added.
11. Invert the bag and add the medication through the medication addition port.
12. Remove the needle and cleanse the medication addition port.
13. Invert the bag several times and place an administration set into it.
14. Bleed the air out of the administration set and attach a 1-inch, 18-gauge needle.
15. Cleanse the medication port on the administration set of the already established IV line and insert the needle (see Figure 3–6).

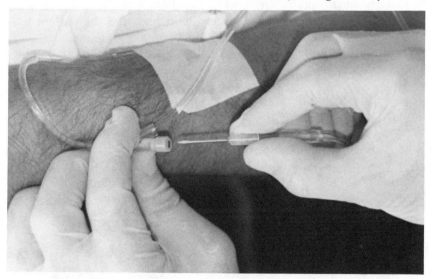

Figure 3–6   Cleanse the medication port and insert the needle.

16. Tape the needle securely.
17. Adjust the flow rate of the piggyback infusion to the desired dose. (see Figure 3–7).

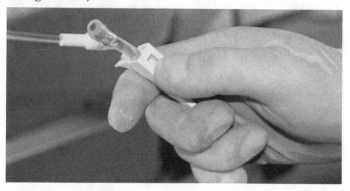

Figure 3–7   Adjust the flow rate to deliver the appropriate dosage.

18. Label the bag for emergency department personnel.
19. Confirm establishment of the infusion.
20. Closely monitor the patient for the desired therapeutic effects as well as any undesired side effects.

Endotracheal Administration

The endotracheal route is very effective and often forgotten in the emergency setting. When an IV cannot be established, and the patient is in dire need of lidocaine, naloxone, atropine, or epinephrine, which may be the case in cardiac arrest, these drugs may be instilled via the endotracheal tube. The rate of absorption is as fast as IV administration. Consider the following:

A patient is encountered in ventricular fibrillation and is immediately countershocked. The patient converts to an improved rhythm with a fair pulse. An IV line cannot be immediately established, however. The patient begins to have frequent multifocal premature ventricular contractions. Lidocaine can now be administered down the endotracheal tube to stabilize the rhythm until a peripheral line can be established.

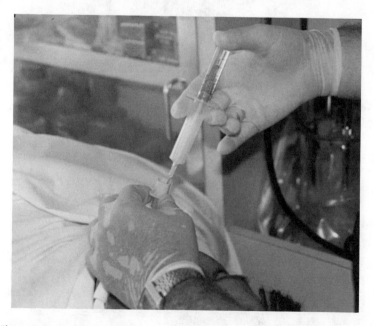

Figure 3–8 Instill the medication down the endotracheal tube and resume ventilations.

The procedure is as follows:

1. Receive the order.
2. Confirm the order and write it down.
3. Prepare the prefilled medication syringe and don gloves.
4. Examine the ampule of medication, reconfirming that it is correct. Quickly hold it up to light and inspect for discoloration or particles in the solution. Do not administer if foreign bodies are present or if discolored.
5. Hyperventilate the patient in anticipation of administration.
6. Remove the bag-valve-mask unit and inject the medication down the tube (see Figure 3–8).
7. Replace the bag-valve-mask unit and resume ventilation.
8. Monitor the patient for the desired therapeutic effect and any possible undesired side effects.

Intraosseous Injection

It is often difficult to establish an IV line in children younger than 2 years of age. In instances in which an IV cannot be established, and the child needs emergency medications or fluids, an intraosseous line can be established. A needle is placed into the proximal tibia, approximately 1 to 3 centimeters below the tibial tuberosity, on the anterior surface. The needle is advanced through the cortex of the bone into the bone marrow cavity. Entry into the marrow cavity is evidenced by a lack of resistance after penetrating the bony cortex, the needle standing upright without support, the ability to aspirate bone marrow into a syringe connected to the needle, or the free flow of the infusion without significant subcutaneous infiltration. Fluids and drugs administered into the marrow cavity quickly enter the circulatory system. The onset of action of drugs administered by this route is similar to IV injection. Drugs that can be administered by this route include the catecholamines, lidocaine, atropine, sodium bicarbonate, as well as fluids. *Intraosseous infusion is only indicated in children younger than 2 years of age and only when an IV line cannot be established.*

The procedure is as follows:

1. Receive the order.
2. Confirm the order and write it down.
3. Prepare the necessary equipment and don gloves:
   - Medication
   - Intravenous fluid
   - Syringe

- Intraosseous needle or 16-to 18-gauge spinal needle
- Provodine iodine preparation

4. Examine the ampule, vial, or syringe of medication or fluid, and make sure it is correct. Also make sure it is not discolored and does not contain any particles. Do not administer if particles are present or if discolored.
5. Locate the anterior tibial tuberosity. Choose a spot approximately 1 to 3 centimeters below.
6. Prepare the area extensively with three provodine iodine preparations in a circular fashion.
7. Replace your gloves with sterile gloves.
8. Take the sterile needle and insert it into the bone at a perpendicular angle or angled slightly inferior. Stop insertion when a lack of resistance is felt (see Figures 3–9 and 3–10).
9. Place a syringe on the needle, and attempt to aspirate a small amount of marrow.
10. If the needle is properly placed (that is, it stands upright without support or you are able to aspirate marrow) attach it to an IV line and the desired fluid. Do not administer IV fluid unless ordered, and then only in doses of 20 milliliters per kilogram.
11. Administer the medication.
12. Remove the syringe. Do not recap the needle. Dispose of the needle and syringe properly.
13. Closely monitor the child for the desired effects as well as any side effects.
14. Secure the intraosseous needle before movement of the child.

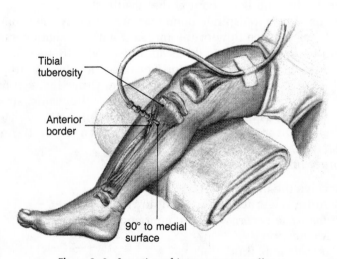

Figure 3–9 Insertion of intraosseous needle.

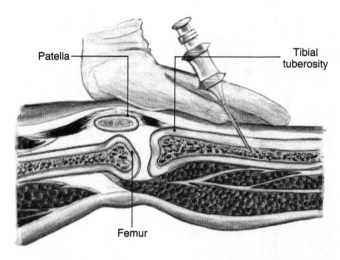

Patella

Tibial
tuberosity

Femur

Figure 3–10   Intraosseous needle properly in place.

Inhalational Administration

Many medications used in the treatment of respiratory emergencies are administered by inhalation. The most common example of this is oxygen. In addition, there are medications that are designed to be administered into the respiratory tree. The most common of these are the bronchodilators. These include metaproterenol (Alupent®), racemic epinephrine, isotharine (Bronkosol®), and albuterol (Ventolin®). By administering these drugs directly into the respiratory tree they can quickly reach their site of action with minimal absorption delays.

The following are three commonly used methods for administering these medications:

Metered Dose Inhalers.   Metered dose inhalers are aerosolized forms of the medication in a small canister. Most bronchodilators are supplied in this form. Many patients have these at home and use them routinely. The canister is attached to a mouthpiece. The patient places his or her lips around the mouthpiece, begins to inhale, and presses the canister. When the canister is pressed, a metered amount of the drug is delivered in aerosol form. The amount of drug delivered is accurate and limited. Metered dose inhalers are designed for single-patient use (see Figure 3–11).

Spinhaler®, Rotohaler®.   These commercial devices are designed for patients who have difficulty operating the metered dose inhalers. Special capsules are placed in the device. When inhaled the capsules release medication that is delivered to the respiratory tree (see Figure 3–12).

Small-volume Nebulizer.   Small-volume nebulizers, also called updraft or hand-held nebulizers, are the most commonly used method of admin-

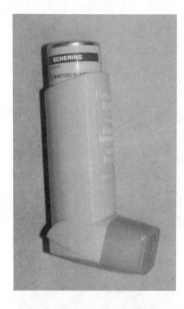

Figure 3–11   Metered dose inhaler.

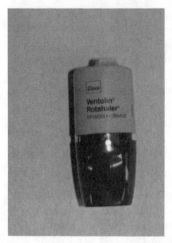

Figure 3–12   Rotohaler.

istering inhaled medications in the emergency setting. The nebulizer has a chamber into which a solution of the medication, usually diluted with 2 to 3 milliliters of sterile saline, is placed. Oxygen or compressed air is blown past the chamber causing the medication to be aerosolized. The patient inhales the aerosolized medication with each breath. This method of bronchodilator administration is advantageous because it delivers supplemental oxygen, delivers the medication over a 5- to 10-minute interval, and is supplied in single-dose ampules (see Figures 3–13 and 3–14).

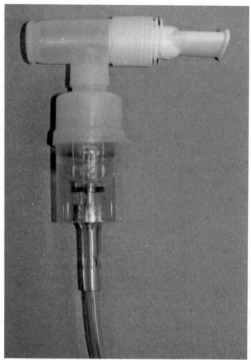

Figure 3–13 Small volume nebulizer.

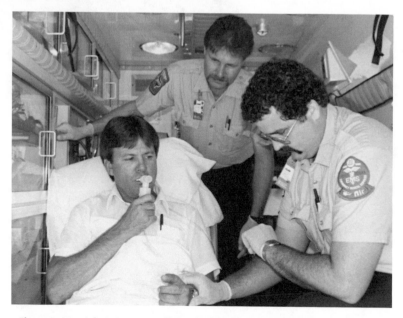

Figure 3–14 Administration of bronchodilators in EMS has become a common procedure.

SUMMARY

It is essential that acute care personnel be competent with all of the medication routes used in emergency medicine. These skills can be developed only after repeated practice in the classroom and the clinical setting. It is important to be familiar with all of the medications used in routine prehospital care in your system and the routes by which they are administered. If there is any doubt concerning an order or an administration route, consult the medical control physician or a drug reference source. Each time you administer a medication you should assure you have met each of the five "rights" of medication administration. These are the following:

1. Right patient
2. Right medication
3. Right dose
4. Right route
5. Right time

This book is not a substitute for a rigorous classroom instruction session on medication adminstration. It is purely designed as a teaching aid for the student and as a reference source for others.

4

DRUG DOSAGE
CALCULATIONS

INTRODUCTION

Administration of the correct drug dosage is essential to proper medical care. Medications used in emergency medicine are available from many different manufacturers, many in different strengths, volumes, and containers. It is important to be familiar with the common emergency drug preparations. In addition, all personnel should be able to prepare the correct medication dose quickly from available ampules or vials regardless of drug concentration or volume.

Familiarity with the systems of measurement frequently used in medicine, especially the metric system, is essential. Conversion from one system to another is often required.

In this chapter, common mathematical operations required to complete dosage calculations as well as several formulas are presented.

SYSTEM OF WEIGHTS AND MEASURES

The metric system is the principal system of weights and measures used in pharmacology. Tradition has caused some apothecaries' weights and measures to endure, however. The metric system is used worldwide as the standard system of weights and measures in both science and medicine. In recent years the U.S. government has begun the arduous transition from the English system to the metric system.

The metric system is a system of weights and measures devised by the French. The metric system is based on the unit 10. All units were either 10 times larger or 1/10 as large as the next unit. Because the metric system is based on 10, the conversion from one unit to another is fairly simple. The change from one set of units to another requires moving only a decimal point.

In making physical descriptions, three things need to be measured: mass, length, and volume. **Mass** is the quantity of matter present in a given substance. **Length** is the distance between two points. **Volume** is the space occupied by a given substance. The metric system has three fundamental units for the measurement of mass, length, and volume. The fundamental unit used for measuring mass is the **gram**. The fundamental unit used for measuring length is the **meter**. And the fundamental unit used for measuring volume is the **liter**. All other metric units used to describe length, mass, and volume are derivatives of these three fundamental, or base, units. Instead of using a large number of zeros, a person making metric conversions can simply change the prefix. Common metric system prefixes include the following:

$$\text{kilo-} = 1000 \text{ (k)}$$

$$\text{hecto-} = 100 \text{ (h)}$$

$$\text{deka-} = 10 \text{ (D)}$$

$$\text{Fundamental unit} = 1 \text{ (gram, liter, or meter)}$$

$$\text{deci-} = 1/10 \text{ (d)}$$

$$\text{centi-} = 1/100 \text{ (c)}$$

$$\text{milli-} = 1/1000 \text{ (m)}$$

$$\text{micro-} = 1/1,100,000 \text{ (}\mu\text{)}$$

The following prefixes are most frequently encountered: kilo-, centi-, milli-, and micro-.

Metric Conversions

To change a prefix, simply move the decimal point. Common examples of metric conversions follow:

$$1000 \text{ liters} = 1 \text{ kiloliter}$$

$$1000 \text{ grams} = 1 \text{ kilogram}$$

$$1/1000 \text{ gram} = 1 \text{ milligram (0.001 gram} = 1.0 \text{ milligram)}$$

$$1/100 \text{ meter} = 1 \text{ centimeter (0.01 meter} = 1.0 \text{ centimeter)}$$

Most of us learned only the English system of measurement while in school. To bring the metric system into perspective, the following are some common conversions with which we need to be familiar:

1 centimeter = 0.39 inches

1 meter = 39.37 inches

1 liter = 1.05 quarts

1 kilogram = 2.2 pounds

2.54 centimeter = 1.0 inch

Occasionally, orders will be received for certain drugs in the old apothecaries' system. The most common apothecary measure likely to be seen is the *grain*. Many physicians still routinely prescribe some medications, especially analgesics, in grains. Because most emergency drugs are most likely in metric measures, a conversion is required. The conversion is as follows:

1 grain = 60 milligrams

thus

¼ grain = 15 milligrams

Another conversion often used in medicine is between cubic centimeters and milliliters. One milliliter of water occupies 1 cubic centimeter of space. Thus:

1 cubic centimeter (cm³) = 1 milliliter (ml)

The term "cubic centimeter" is falling into disuse, with milliliter being the preferred term. Occasionally both may be seen, however.

Familiarity with the metric system, and its conversions, is essential. The following practice problems should be mastered before moving to the next section.

In addition to the trend in medicine toward the metric system, we are also seeing the switch from the use of the Fahrenheit system of temperature measurement to the Celsius system. The Celsius system is based on the physical properties of water. The freezing point was designated 0°C, which is 32°F. The boiling point of water was designated 100°C, which is 212°F. Thus, normal body temperature is either 98.6°F or 37°C. The conversion is as follows:

From Fahrenheit to Celsius:

(Degrees F − 32) × 0.556 = Degrees C

From Celsius to Fahrenheit:

$$(\text{Degrees C} \times 1.8) + 32 = \text{Degrees F}$$

Example:

$$(98.6 - 32) \times 0.556 = 37°C$$
$$37 \times 1.8 = 66.6 + 32 = 98.6°F$$

PRACTICE PROBLEMS

Convert the following:

1. 2 kilograms = _____grams
2. 300 milligrams = _____grams
3. 1.5 grams = _____milligrams
4. 500 milliliters = _____liters
5. 1 liter = _____milliliters
6. ½ grain = _____milligrams
7. 90 milligrams = _____grains
8. 175°F = _____°C
9. 10°C = _____°F
10. 15 centimeters = _____inches
11. 2 inches = _____centimeters
12. 187 pounds = _____kilograms
13. 95 kilograms = _____pounds
14. 231 pounds = _____kilograms
15. 35 kilograms = _____pounds

(Answers can be found on page 48.)

DRUG CALCULATIONS

Each textbook has its own method of presenting the process of drug calculations. This text is no different. Most drug calculations required in prehospital care are generally quite similar. They range from simple parenteral calculations to more elaborate infusion calculations integrating time intervals into the process. When making a calculation, the following information will normally be available:

Desired Dose. The desired dose is the quantity of medication or fluid that the physician wants the patient to receive. This is usually expressed in milligrams, grams, or grains.

Concentration of Drug on Hand. The concentration of the drug on hand is the amount of the drug present in the ampule or vial. This is usually expressed in milligrams, grams, or grains.

Volume of Drug on Hand. The volume of the drug on hand is the amount of fluid within the ampule or vial into which the drug is dissolved. This is usually represented in milliliters.

Based on the information presented earlier, the calculation of the volume of the drug to be administered to the patient can be made. The following formula represents this relationship:

$$\text{VOLUME TO BE ADMINISTERED (X)} = \frac{\text{(VOLUME ON HAND) (DESIRED DOSE)}}{\text{(CONCENTRATION ON HAND)}}$$

Example 1

A physician wants 5 milligrams of parenteral Valium® administered to a patient. The Valium ampule contains 10 milligrams of Valium in 2 milliliters of solvent. The following calculation must then be made (see Figure 4–1):

$$\text{VOLUME ADMIN (X)} = \frac{\text{VOLUME ON HAND (2 ml) DESIRED DOSE (5 mg)}}{\text{CONCENTRATION ON HAND (10 mg)}}$$

To solve, multiply:

$$X = \frac{(2 \text{ ml})(5 \text{ mg})}{10 \text{ mg})}$$

Thus:

$$X = \frac{10}{10}$$

Then:

$$X = 1 \text{ ml}$$

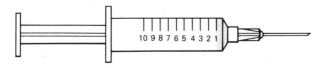

Figure 4–1   Correct dosage is 1 milliliter.

Example 2

A physician wants 75 milligrams of lidocaine administered to a patient in an IV bolus. The drug is supplied in a prefilled syringe containing 100 milligrams of lidocaine in 5 milliliters of solvent. Calculate the number of milliliters to be administered. The calculation is as follows (see Figure 4–2):

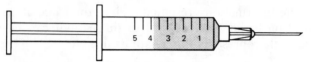

Figure 4–2   Correct dosage is 3.75 milliliters.

$$X = \frac{(5 \text{ ml})(75 \text{ mg})}{(100 \text{ mg})}$$

Thus:

$$X = \frac{375}{100}$$

Then:

$$X = 3.75 \text{ ml}$$

This formula holds true for all of the drug calculations routinely used in emergency medicine, but it works only if all of the measurements are in the same units.

Variations on a Theme

The formula presented earlier is useful for calculating the infusion rate of IV drips. All that is required is to multiply "X" times the drops per milliliter delivered by your set. The end result will be the number of drops per minute that needs to be delivered.

Example 3

A physician wants 2 milligrams per minute of lidocaine administered to a patient. She orders 2 grams of lidocaine to be placed into 500 milliliters of 5% dextrose in water. A minidrip infusion set that delivers 60 drops per milliliter is being used. The problem can be solved as follows (see Figure 4–3):

$$\frac{(500 \text{ ml})(2 \text{ mg/min})}{(2000 \text{ mg})} \times 60 \text{ drops/ml} = X \text{ drops/min}$$

Then:

$$\frac{(1000)}{(2000)} = 0.5 \times 60 \text{ drops/ml} = 30 \text{ drops/min}$$

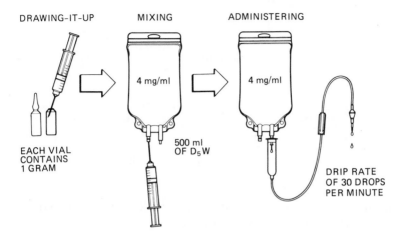

DRAWING-IT-UP   MIXING   ADMINISTERING

4 mg/ml

4 mg/ml

EACH VIAL
CONTAINS
1 GRAM

500 ml
OF D₅W

DRIP RATE
OF 30 DROPS
PER MINUTE

Figure 4–3 Correct dosage is 30 drops/minute.

Other Calculations

Sometimes an order will be received to administer a drug to a patient based on the patient's weight. The drug dosage must then be calculated based on the patient's weight. This can then be plugged into the formula.

Example 4

A physician wants a patient to receive 5 milligrams per kilogram body weight of Bretylol®. The patient weighs 220 pounds. The Bretylol® is supplied in ampules containing 500 milligrams in 10 milliliters. How many milliliters of the drug should be administered?

To solve this problem, two preliminary calculations are required. First, the patient's weight must be converted to kilograms. Then, the patient's weight, in kilograms, must be multiplied by the number of milligrams per kilogram that is to be delivered. The calculation goes as follows (see Figure 4–4):

1. Convert pounds to kilograms:

$$\frac{220 \text{ lb}}{2.2 \text{ lb/kg}} = 100 \text{ kg}$$

2. Calculate the desired dose:

$$100 \text{ kgrams} \times 5 \text{ milligrams/kilogram} = 500 \text{ milligrams}$$

3. Calculate the volume to be administered using the formula:

$$X = \frac{(10 \text{ ml})(500 \text{ mg})}{(500 \text{ mg})}$$

Then:

$$X = \frac{(5000)}{(500)} = 10 \text{ ml}$$

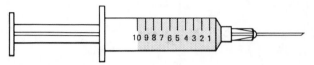

Figure 4–4   Correct dosage is 10 milliliters.

One additional calculation that is often made is to calculate the rate of infusion of an IV fluid not containing any medication.

Example 5

The emergency physician wants a 1-liter bag of lactated Ringer's to be infused into a patient over 2 hours. The IV administration set delivers 10 drops per milliliter. How many drops per minute should be infused?

To solve this problem, the formula presented earlier is not used. Instead, the volume of fluid should be divided by the number of minutes over which the fluid is to be administered. Then, that value is multiplied by the rate of the set.

1. Convert hours to minutes:

$$2 \text{ hr} \times 60 \text{ min/hr} = 120 \text{ min}$$

2. Divide the volume of fluid by the number of minutes:

$$\frac{1000 \text{ ml}}{120 \text{ min}} = 8.3 \text{ ml/min}$$

3. To determine the number of drops per minute:

$$8.3 \text{ ml/min} \times 10 \text{ drops/ml} = 83 \text{ drops/min}$$

PRACTICE PROBLEMS

1. A physician wants you to administer 50 milligrams of lidocaine. Lidocaine is supplied in 5-milliliter ampules containing 100 milligrams of the drug. How many milliliters should you administer?
2. You are ordered to give a patient 1 mEq of sodium bicarbonate per kilogram of body weight. The patient weighs 77 pounds. If sodium

bicarbonate is supplied in 50-milliliter syringes containing 50 mEq of the drug, how many milliliters should you administer?

3. You are to give a patient 0.8 milligrams of Narcan®. Narcan® is supplied in 1-milliliter ampules containing 0.4 milligram of the drug. How many milliliters should you administer?

4. You are to administer 3 milligrams per minute of lidocaine in an infusion. The physician asks you to place 1 gram of lidocaine in 1 liter of 5% dextrose in water. If you use a minidrip set, which delivers 60 drops per milliliter, how many drops per minute would you deliver?

5. You are to administer 0.4 milligrams of 1:1000 epinephrine. Epinephrine 1:1000 contains 1 milligram of the drug in 1 milliliter of solvent. How many milliliters should you deliver?

6. You are to administer 1 liter of 0.9% sodium chloride over a 4-hour period. If you use an infusion set that delivers 10 drops per milliliter, how many drops per minute would you infuse?

7. You are to administer 5 milligrams per kilogram of Bretylol®. Bretylol® is supplied in ampules containing 500 milligrams of the drug in 10 milliliters of solvent. If the patient weighs 165 pounds, how many milliliters would you give?

8. A physician orders you to administer ½ of a gram of calcium chloride to a patient in cardiac arrest. If calcium chloride comes in a 10-milliliter syringe containing 1000 milligrams, how many milliliters would you administer?

9. You are ordered to administer 2 liters of lactated Ringer's over 6 hours. If the administration set you are going to use delivers 10 drops per milliliter, how many drops per minute should you infuse?

10. You are to deliver 150 micrograms per kilogram per minute of Intropin® to a patient. The patient weighs 110 pounds. You are ordered to place 4 ampules of Intropin® into 500 milliliters of 5% dextrose. Each ampule contains 200 milligrams. Using a minidrip set, which delivers 60 drops per milliliter, how many drops per minute should you infuse?

(Answers can be found on page 48.)

SUMMARY

Drug calculations and the metric system will become easier with experience. It is a process that is used throughout clinical training as well as every day on the job. The fundamental skills presented in this chapter must be mastered before confidence in the system can be developed. Practice problems are always helpful.

PRACTICE PROBLEM ANSWERS

Page 42

1. 2000 grams
2. 0.3 gram
3. 1500 milligrams
4. 0.5 liter
5. 1000 milliliters
6. 30 milligrams
7. 1.5 grains
8. 79.5°C
9. 50°F
10. 5.9 inches
11. 5 centimeters
12. 85 kilograms
13. 209 pounds
14. 105 kilograms
15. 15.9 kilograms

Page 46

1. 2.5 milliliters
2. 35 milliliters
3. 2 milliliters
4. 180 drops per minute
5. 0.4 milliliter
6. 41.6 drops per minute
7. 7.5 milliliters
8. 5 milliliters
9. 55.6 drops per minute
10. 28.1 drops per minute

Additional practice problems can be found in Appendix F.

5

FLUIDS, ELECTROLYTES, AND IV THERAPY

INTRODUCTION

One of the most important aspects of prehospital care is the administration of IV fluids and electrolytes. There are two major reasons for administering intravenous fluids during the prehospital phase of emergency medical care. The first is to replace immediately intravascular blood volume. The second is to provide an easily accessible route for the administration of lifesaving emergency drugs.

FLUIDS

The most abundant substance in the human body is **water**. Approximately 60% of the total body weight is water, which is located within two fluid compartments (or spaces). The largest of these fluid compartments is the **intracellular** space. The intracellular compartment includes all fluids found within the cells. Three-fourths of all body water is within the intracellular space. The remaining water can be found outside of the cell membrane in the **extracellular** fluid compartment. There are two major components of the extracellular fluid compartment. The first is **intravascular** fluid. Intravascular fluid is found within the blood vessels and outside of the cell membrane. The other component of the extracellular fluid compartment is the **interstitial** fluid. The interstitial fluid is that fluid found outside the cell membrane, yet not within any defined blood vessels. The relationship of the various fluid compartments is illustrated as follows:

EXTRACELLULAR FLUID .... 15% of Total Body Weight
    (Interstitial Fluid = 10.5% of Total Body Weight)
    (Intravascular Fluid = 4.5% of Total Body Weight)
INTRACELLULAR FLUID .... 45% of Total Body Weight

TOTAL BODY WATER .... 60% of Total Body Weight

INTERNAL ENVIRONMENT

The internal environment is the extracellular fluid discussed earlier. The extracellular fluid bathes each body cell. There is an important balance that must be maintained regarding the internal environment. Whenever one aspect of the internal environment deviates from normal, as frequently occurs in injury and illness, the body will immediately respond and return to normal. The body's tendency to maintain all of its physiological activities in proper balance, including the internal environment, is called **homeostasis**.

ELECTROLYTES

In addition to the body fluids, there are also important chemicals that are required for life. These chemicals are divided into two main classes: **electrolytes** and **nonelectrolytes**. Chemicals that take on an electrical charge when placed into water are called electrolytes. Chemicals that do not take on electrical charge are called nonelectrolytes. All electrolytes are measured in quantities called milliequivalents (mEq). Sodium bicarbonate, a common emergency drug, is an electrolyte. When placed into water, it quickly divides into charged particles or **ions**. All dosages of sodium bicarbonate are calculated in milliequivalents.

Certain electrolytes, when dissolved in water, take on a positive charge. These are called **cations**. Examples of common cations include sodium (Na^+), potassium (K^+), magnesium (Mg^{++}), and calcium (Ca^{++}). Electrolytes that take on a negative charge are called **anions**. Examples of anions found within the body include chlorine (Cl^-), bicarbonate (HCO_3^-), and most of the organic (carbon based) molecules. In addition to the fluid balance mentioned earlier, electrical neutrality must be carefully maintained between cations and anions.

CELL PHYSIOLOGY

To maintain physiological homeostasis, there must be an exchange of electrolytes and water materials across the membrane of the cell. The cell membrane is very complex. It is said to be **semipermeable**, meaning that it allows certain compounds to pass readily across it while restricting the passage of others. Many materials must pass across the cell membrane including oxygen, carbon dioxide, nutrients, fluids, and electrolytes. There are two major ways to move substances across the cell membrane: **diffusion** and **active transport**. Diffusion is a passive process, whereas active transport requires energy expenditure by the cell (see Figure 5–1).

Diffusion occurs when concentrations of various substances become higher on one side of the semipermeable cell membrane. When this difference occurs, a **gradient** is created. The side of the cell membrane with the higher concentration is said to be **hypertonic** with respect to the other side. Conversely, the side of the membrane with the lower concentration is said to be **hypotonic** in relation to the other (see Figure 5–2).

When both sides of the cell membrane have an equal concentration of the substance in question, the system is said to be **isotonic**. These concepts underpin the rationale for IV therapy. IV fluids with a solute concentration

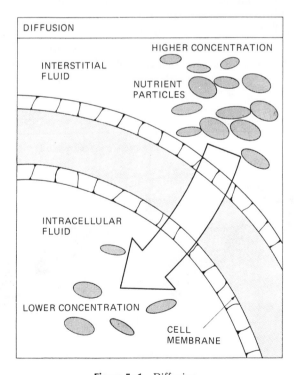

Figure 5–1   Diffusion.

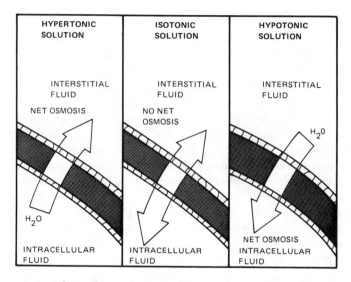

Figure 5–2 Relationship and effects of hypotonic, isotonic, and hypertonic solutions.

less than that of blood are said to be *hypotonic* solutions. An example of a hypotonic solution is 0.45% sodium chloride.

Substances that have a solute concentration equal to that of blood are said to be *isotonic*. Lactated Ringer's and 0.9% sodium chloride are examples of isotonic fluids. An example of a hypertonic solution is 50% dextrose in water. Although not a classical "IV fluid," it plays a major

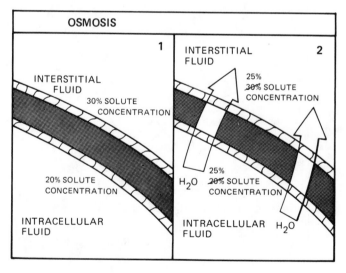

Figure 5–3 Osmosis.

role in prehospital care. One of the most important substances that passes across the cell membrane is water. Water will diffuse readily across the cell membrane from an area of higher water concentration to an area of lesser water concentration. The diffusion of water in this manner is called **osmosis** (see Figure 5–3).

Sometimes it is desirable for the body to maintain a gradient along a cell membrane. This is especially true regarding the ions sodium (Na^+) and potassium (K^+). To sustain life, the concentration of sodium outside the cell membrane must be significantly higher than that inside the cell. Also, the concentration of potassium must be maintained at a much higher level within the cell. To maintain the gradient, the sodium must be pumped out of the cell and potassium must be pumped into the cell. Both of these processes require energy. This is an example of active transport.

BLOOD

One of the most important aspects of the extracellular fluid, and thus the internal environment, is blood. Blood is responsible for transport of oxygen (O_2) to cells and carbon dioxide (CO_2) from cells.

There are two major aspects of blood: fluid and cells. The fluid in which all of the blood cells are suspended is called **plasma** (see Figure 5–4).

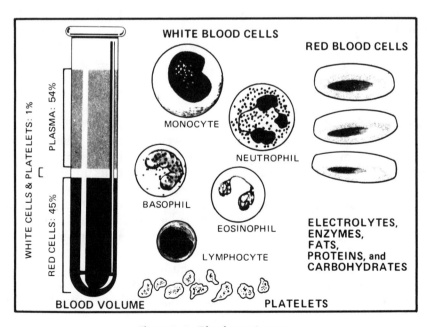

Figure 5–4 Blood constituents.

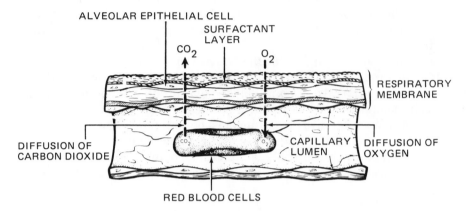

ALVEOLUS

Figure 5–5   The red blood cell.

There are three major classes of blood cells. The first are the red blood cells or **erythrocytes** (see Figure 5–5). Erythrocytes contain an important iron-containing protein called **hemoglobin**. Hemoglobin is responsible for the transport of oxygen and carbon dioxide.

A significant percentage of blood, approximately 45 percent, is red blood cells. The percentage of red blood cells present is referred to as the **hematocrit**. The second type of cells found in the blood is the white blood cells or **leukocytes**. The leukocytes are responsible for combating infection. The last type of blood cell present are the platelets or **thrombocytes**, responsible for blood clotting.

IV THERAPY

As mentioned earlier, there are two major indications for IV therapy. The first is to replace fluid losses, which may occur as a result of hemorrhage caused by trauma or from severe diarrhea, vomiting, heat exhaustion, and burns. It is best to replace the fluid losses with intravenous fluids of similar isotonicity.

There are two major classes of IV fluids: colloids and crystalloids. **Colloids** contain compounds of high molecular weight, usually proteins, which do not readily diffuse across the cell membrane. Common examples of colloids include **Plasmanate®** and **Dextran®**.

Crystalloids contain only water and electrolytes. These substances will all readily diffuse across the cell membrane. Common crystalloids used in emergency medicine include **lactated Ringer's, 5% dextrose in water,** and **sodium chloride**, among others.

In cases of hypovolemic shock, characterized by significant blood loss, experts think colloids are the fluid of choice because they remain in the intravascular space, thus increasing the overall circulating volume. Despite the seeming advantage of colloids over crystalloids in the management of hypovolemia, however, they are rarely used in the prehospital phase of emergency medical care. Their high cost and short shelf life are the major reasons. When colloids are not available, the crystalloid lactated Ringer's is the IV fluid of choice for the management of most hypovolemic states. Lactated Ringer's is isotonic. Electrolytes are present in approximately the same concentration as those in the blood.

The second reason for initiating an IV infusion in the field is to provide a route for the administration of drugs. Although most IV fluids will work, 5% dextrose in water is usually chosen.

The following IV fluids are most frequently used in prehospital emergency care (see Table 5–1).

Plasma Protein Fraction (Plasmanate®)

Description

Plasmanate is a protein-containing colloid used in the treatment of hypovolemic shock. The principal protein in Plasmanate is serum human albumin suspended in a saline solvent. Because of the high molecular weight of the protein, Plasmanate tends to remain in the intravascular space for an extended period.

Plasmanate is quite expensive and has a very short shelf life. Although rarely used in the prehospital phase of emergency medical care, Plasmanate is preferred by some emergency specialists in the management of hypovolemic states, especially burn shock. After a patient sustains a severe burn, fluid is lost from the blood into the surrounding tissue. Plasmanate, because it remains in the circulating blood volume, is effective in maintaining adequate blood volume and blood pressure. It is usually used in combination with lactated Ringer's.

Indication

- Hypovolemic shock, especially burn shock

Contraindications

There are no major contraindications to Plasmanate when used in the treatment of life-threatening hypovolemic states.

TABLE 5–1 Approximate Ionic Concentrations (mEq/l) and Calories per Liter

	Ionic Concentrations (mEq/l)					Calories per liter	Osmolarity[a] (mOsm/l)	pH Range[b]
	Sodium	Potassium	Calcium	Chloride	Lactate			
5% Dextrose Injection, USP	0	0	0	0	0	170	252	3.5–6.5
10% Dextrose Injection, USP	0	0	0	0	0	340	505	3.5–6.5
0.9% Sodium Chloride Injection, USP	154	0	0	154	0	0	308	4.5–7.0
Sodium Lactate Injection, USP (M/6 Sodium Lactate)	167	0	0	0	167	54	334	6.0–7.3
2.5% Dextrose & 0.45% Sodium Chloride Injection, USP	77	0	0	77	0	85	280	3.5–6.0
5% Dextrose & 0.2% Sodium Chloride Injection, USP	34	0	0	34	0	170	321	3.5–6.0
5% Dextrose & 0.33% Sodium Chloride Injection, USP	56	0	0	56	0	170	365	3.5–6.0
5% Dextrose & 0.45% Sodium Chloride Injection, USP	77	0	0	77	0	170	406	3.5–6.0
5% Dextrose & 0.9% Sodium Chloride Injection, USP	154	0	0	154	0	170	560	3.5–6.0
10% Dextrose & 0.9% Sodium Chloride Injection, USP	154	0	0	154	0	340	813	3.5–6.0
Ringer's Injection, USP	147.5	4	4.5	156	0	0	309	5.0–7.5
Lactated Ringer's Injection, USP	130	4	3	109	28	9	273	6.0–7.5
5% Dextrose in Ringer's Injection	147.5	4	4.5	156	0	170	561	3.5–6.5
Lactated Ringer's with 5% Dextrose	130	4	3	109	28	180	525	4.0–6.5

[a]Normal physiolical isotonicity range is approximately 280–310 mOsm/l. Administration of substantially hypotonic solutions may cause hemolysis and administration of substantially hypertonic solutions may cause vein damage.

[b]pH ranges are USP for applicable solution, corporate specification for non-USP solutions.
(Adapted with permission from Travenol Laboratories, Inc., Deerfield, Illinois)

Precautions

It is important to monitor constantly the response of the patient and adjust the rate of infusion accordingly. Monitor patient for elevated blood pressure and pulmonary edema during and following Plasmanate administration.

Dosage

The Plasmanate infusion rate should be titrated according to the patient's hemodynamic response. In the management of shock secondary to burns, physician's orders regarding the rate of administration must be closely followed. Standard formulas for IV fluid administration have been developed. The base station physician will use these in judging the correct rate of intravenous administration.

Routes

Plasmanate is given by intravenous infusion.

How Supplied

Plasmanate is supplied in 250 and 500 milliliter bottles of a 5% solution. An administration is usually attached.

Dextran®

Description

Dextran is a colloid differing significantly from Plasmanate® or any of the other plasma protein fractions. Instead of proteins, Dextran contains chains of sugars that are approximately the same molecular weight as serum albumin. Thus, because of their large molecular size, they remain within the circulating blood volume for an extended period. Although not as effective as Plasmanate, Dextran has proved effective as an adjunctive aid in the management of hypovolemic shock. Because Dextran is secreted through the urine, urine output is usually maintained with the administration of Dextran. *A major drawback to the use of Dextran is that it coats the red blood cells, thus preventing accurate blood typing and thus possibly hindering administration of whole blood if required.*

Indication

- Hypovolemic shock

Contraindications

Dextran should not be administered to patients who have a known hypersensitivity to the drug. It should also not be administered to patients who are receiving anticoagulants as it significantly retards blood clotting.

Precautions

Severe anaphylactic reactions have been known to occur following the administration of Dextran. The patient should be closely monitored, and emergency resuscitative drugs should be readily available. Because of the sodium content, it is important to watch for possible circulatory overload presenting as edema and elevated blood pressure.

It is preferrable to use crystalloid solutions, such as lactated Ringer's, rather than Dextran, in the management of profound hypovolemic shock.

A tube of blood should be drawn before administering Dextran for blood typing at the hospital.

Dosage

The dosage of Dextran is titrated according to the patient's physiological response. In the management of burn shock it is especially important to follow standard fluid resuscitation regimens to prevent possible circulatory overload.

Routes

Dextran is given only by intravenous infusion.

How Supplied

Dextran is supplied in two molecular weights. Dextran 40 has an average molecular weight of approximately 40,000. Dextran 40 is secreted by the kidneys much more readily than the higher molecular weight form, Dextran 70 (molecular weight = 70,000). The higher molecular weight form tends to be broken down into glucose instead of being secreted in the Dextran form, as occurs with Dextran 40. The decision on which type of Dextran to use in prehospital care rests with the system medical director.

Dextran 40 and Dextran 70 are supplied in 250- and 500-milliliter bottles.

Hetastarch (Hespan®)

Description

Hetastarch is an artificial colloid differing from both Plasmanate® and Dextran®. Hetastarch is derived from amylopectin and chemically resembles glycogen. The average molecular weight is approximately 450,000, which gives it colloidal properties similar to that of human albumin. Intravenous infusion of hetastarch results in plasma volume expansion slightly greater than the amount infused.

Because the colloidal properties of hetastarch are quite similar to those of human albumin, it has proved effective in the management of hypovolemic shock, especially burn shock. It does not appear to share the blood typing problems seen with Dextran.

Indication

- Hypovolemic shock, especially burn shock

Contraindications

There are no major contraindications to hetastarch when used in the management of life-threatening hypovolemic states.

Precautions

It is important to monitor constantly the response of the patient and adjust the rate of infusion accordingly. Monitor the patient for signs of pulmonary edema and elevated blood pressure during and following hetastarch administration.

Large volumes of hetastarch may alter the body's coagulation mechanism. Hetastarch should be used with caution in the patients receiving anticoagulants.

Dosage

The hetastarch infusion rate should be titrated according to the patient's hemodynamic response. In the management of burn shock, physician's orders regarding the rate of administration must be closely followed. Standard formulas for colloid administration to burn patients have been developed. It is important to remember that a fall in blood pressure in burn shock occurs much later than with hemorrhagic causes.

Route

Hetastarch is given by intravenous infusion.

How Supplied

Sterile 6% hetastarch in 0.9% sodium chloride is supplied in 500-milliliter bottles.

Lactated Ringer's (Hartman's Solution)

Description

Lactated Ringer's solution is the most frequently used IV fluid in the management of hypovolemic shock. It is an isotonic crystalloid solution. The electrolytes and their concentrations are as follows:

Sodium (Na^+) . . . . .130 mEq/liter
Potassium (K^+) . . . . 4 mEq/liter
Calcium (Ca^{++}) . . . . 3 mEq/liter
Chlorine (Cl^-) . . . . .109 mEq/liter

In addition to the electrolytes mentioned earlier, lactated Ringer's contains 28 mEq of lactate (lactic acid), which acts as a buffer.

Indication

- Hypovolemic shock

Contraindications

Lactated Ringer's should not be used in patients with congestive heart failure or renal failure.

Precautions

Patients receiving lactated Ringer's should be monitored to prevent circulatory overload.

Dosage

Crystalloids, such as lactated Ringer's, diffuse out of the intravascular space and into the surrounding tissues in less than an hour. Thus, it is often necessary to replace a liter of lost blood with 3 to 4 liters of lactated Ringer's.

In severe hypovolemic shock, lactated Ringer's should be infused through large-bore (14- or 16-gauge) IV cannulas. These infusions should be administered "wide open" until a systolic blood pressure of approximately 100 millimeters of mercury is achieved. When this blood pressure is attained, the infusion should be reduced to about 100 milliliters per hour. If the blood pressure falls again, then the infusion rate should be increased and adjusted accordingly. Adjunctive devices, such as the PASG and extremity elevation, should be used in the management of severe hypovolemic shock.

How Supplied

Lactated Ringer's is supplied in 250-, 500-, and 1000-milliliter bags and bottles.

5% Dextrose in Water (D₅W)

Description

When vigorous fluid replacement is not indicated, 5% dextrose in water (D_5W) is frequently used. D_5W is ideal for providing a lifeline for the administration of intravenous drugs. D_5W is hypotonic, which prevents circulatory overload in patients with congestive heart failure.

Indications

- IV access for emergency drugs
- For dilution of concentrated drugs for intravenous infusion

Contraindications

D_5W should not be used as a fluid replacement for hypovolemic states.

Precautions

As with any IV fluid, it is important to watch for signs of circulatory overload when administering D_5W.

When treating hypoglycemia, it is imperative that a tube of blood is drawn before administering D_5W or 50% dextrose.

Dosage

D_5W is usually administered through a minidrip (60 drops/milliliter) set at a rate of "to keep open" (TKO).

How Supplied

D_5W is supplied in bags and bottles of 50, 100, 150, 250, 500, and 1000 milliliters.

10% Dextrose in Water (D₁₀W)

Description

Ten percent dextrose in water ($D_{10}W$) is a hypertonic solution. Like D_5W, $D_{10}W$ is used only when vigorous fluid replacement is not indicated. $D_{10}W$ has twice as much carbohydrate as does D_5W, which makes it of use in the management of hypoglycemia.

Indications

- Hypoglycemia
- Neonatal resuscitation

Contraindications

$D_{10}W$ should not be used as a fluid replacement for hypovolemic states.

Precautions

As with any IV fluid, it is important to be alert for signs of circulatory overload.

When treating hypoglycemia, it is imperative that a tube of blood is drawn before administering $D_{10}W$ or 50% dextrose.

Dosage

The administration rate of $D_{10}W$ will usually be dependent on the patient's condition.

How Supplied

$D_{10}W$ is supplied in bottles and bags of 50, 100, 150, 250, 500, and 1000 milliliters.

0.9% Sodium Chloride (Normal Saline)

Description

The use of 0.9% sodium chloride, or normal saline as it is often called, has several applications in emergency medicine. Normal saline contains 154 milliequivalents per liter of sodium ions (Na^+) and approximately 154 milliequivalents per liter of chloride (Cl^-) ions. Because the concentration of sodium is near that of blood, the solution is considered isotonic.

Normal saline is especially useful in heat stroke, heat exhaustion, and diabetic ketoacidosis.

Indications

- Heat-related problems (heat exhaustion, heat stroke, and so on)
- Freshwater drowning
- Hypovolemia
- Diabetic ketoacidosis

Contraindications

The use of 0.9% sodium chloride should not be considered in patients with congestive heart failure as circulatory overload can be easily induced.

Precautions

Normal saline contains only sodium and chloride. When large amounts of normal saline are administered, it is quite possible for other important physiological electrolytes to become depleted. In cases in which large amounts of fluids may have to be administered, it might be prudent to use lactated Ringer's.

Dosage

The specific situation being treated will dictate the rate in which normal saline will be administered. In severe heat stroke, diabetic ketoacidosis, and freshwater drowning, it is quite likely that you will be called on to administer the fluid quite rapidly. In other cases, it is advisable to administer the fluid at a moderate rate (for example, 100 milliliters per hour).

How Supplied

Normal saline is supplied in 250-, 500-, and 1000-milliliter bags and bottles. Sterile normal saline for irrigation should not be confused with that designed for intravenous administration.

0.45% Sodium Chloride (½ Normal Saline)

Description

One-half normal saline (0.45% sodium chloride) solution is a hypotonic crystalloid solution containing approximately one-half the concentration of sodium and chloride as does blood plasma.

Indication

- Patients with diminished renal or cardiovascular function for which rapid rehydration is not indicated

Contraindications

Cases in which rapid rehydration is indicated.

Precautions

One-half normal saline contains only sodium and chloride. When large amounts of one-half normal saline are administered, it is possible for other important physiological electrolytes to become depleted. In cases in which large amounts of fluids must be administered, it might be prudent to use lactated Ringer's.

Dosage

The specific situation and patient condition will dictate the rate at which one-half normal saline will be administered.

How Supplied

One-half normal saline is supplied in 250-, 500-, and 1000-milliliter bags and bottles.

5% Dextrose in 0.45% Sodium Chloride (D$_5$½NS)

Description

Five percent dextrose in 0.45% sodium chloride (D$_5$½NS) is a versatile fluid. It contains the same amount of sodium and chloride as does one-half normal saline. Dextrose has been added for its nutrient properties, which provides 80 calories per liter.

Indications

- Heat exhaustion
- Diabetic disorders
- For use as a TKO solution in patients with impaired renal or cardio-vascular function.

Contraindication

D$_5$½NS should not be used when rapid fluid resuscitation is indicated.

Precautions

As with any dextrose-containing solution, a blood sample should be drawn before administering D$_5$½NS to patients with suspected cases of hypo-glycemia.

Dosage

The specific situation and patient condition will dictate the rate at which D$_5$½NS should be administered.

How Supplied

D$_5$½NS is supplied in bottles and bags containing 250, 500, and 1000 milliliters of the fluid.

5% Dextrose in 0.9% Sodium Chloride (D₅NS)

Description

Five percent dextrose in 0.9% normal saline is a hypertonic crystalloid to which 5 grams of dextrose per 100 milliliters of fluid has been added for its nutrient properties.

Indications

- Heat-related disorders
- Freshwater drowning
- Hypovolemia
- Peritonitis

Contraindications

D₅NS should not be administered to patients with impaired cardiac or renal function.

Precautions

D₅NS contains only the electrolytes sodium and chloride. When large amounts of fluids must be administered, it might be prudent to use lactated Ringer's solution so as to prevent depletion of the other physiological electrolytes. It is important to draw a blood sample before administering D₅NS in patients with hypoglycemia.

Dosage

The specific situation and patient condition will dictate the rate at which D₅NS is given.

How Supplied

D₅NS is supplied in bags and bottles containing 250, 500, and 1000 milliliters of the solution.

5% Dextrose in Lactated Ringer's (D₅LR)

Description

Five percent dextrose in lactated Ringer's (D₅LR) contains the same concentration of electrolytes as does lactated Ringer's. In addition to the electrolytes, however, 5 grams of dextrose per 100 milliliters of fluid has been added for nutrient properties. This added dextrose causes the solution to be hypertonic.

Indications

- Hypovolemic shock
- Hemmorhagic shock
- Certain cases of acidosis

Contraindications

D_5LR should not be administered to patients with decreased renal or cardiovascular function.

Precautions

Patients receiving D_5LR should be constantly monitored for signs of circulatory overload. It is essential that a blood sample is drawn before administering D_5LR to patients with hypoglycemia.

Dosage

In severe hypovolemic shock D_5LR should be infused through a large-bore catheter (14 or 16 gauge). This infusion should be administered "wide open" until a blood pressure of 100 millimeters of mercury is achieved. When the blood pressure is attained, the infusions should be reduced to 100 milliliters per hour. In other cases, the specific situation and patient condition will dictate the rate of administration.

How Supplied

D_5NS is supplied in bags and bottles containing 250, 500, and 1000 milliliters of the fluid.

INSERTION OF INDWELLING IV CATHETER

One of the earliest stages in the management of an acutely ill or injured patient is the placement of an IV catheter. In trauma cases, an IV catheter will provide access for fluid resuscitation, whereas in medical disorders it will provide a route for drugs that must be given intravenously.

Before inserting an IV catheter, several decisions must be made to ensure the best possible care for the patient. They are the following:

1. **What size catheter should be inserted?**
   When managing patients with trauma who require rapid fluid administration, it is imperative that a large catheter, either 14 or 16 gauge,

be inserted. It is important to remember that patients who are likely to need whole blood on arrival at the hospital require a large-bore catheter.

2. **What type of IV catheter should be inserted?**

    As a rule, an "over the needle" catheter is all that should be used in the prehospital setting. Butterfly catheters are usually too small to administer large amounts of fluids rapidly. Butterfly catheters should be carried for use in children, however. Occasionally, an adult with exceptionally small veins may be encountered and, in this case, a butterfly may be inserted if one of the other types of catheters cannot be placed.

3. **What type of IV fluid should be used?**

    Usually, this decision will be left up to the base station physician. However, it is important to be familiar with the types of fluids that have been discussed in this chapter and anticipate the physician's order.

4. **What type of administration set should be used?**

    There are two general types of IV administration sets. The **macrodrip** or **standard** set delivers in the neighborhood of 10 to 20 drops per milliliter depending on the manufacturer. **Minidrip** or **microdrip** sets deliver anywhere from 50 to 60 drops per milliliter depending on the manufacturer. If you are going to administer a large quantity of fluids, then you should use a macrodrip set. Anytime you are going to administer a drug, you should use a minidrip set. This is especially true for piggyback drug infusions. Many systems also use Buretrol® or Volutrol® sets for administering aminophylline and similar drugs. If your system uses these sets, you should remember them when preparing to administer drugs like aminophylline.

5. **Where should the IV be inserted?**

    Routinely, IV infusions should be started in the larger veins of the forearm. These are usually the most accessible and the least painful for the patient. When these veins are not available, as often occurs in shock and trauma, then any of the other peripheral sites should be attempted. The veins of the leg and the external jugular in the neck are considered peripheral veins. When treating medical or traumatic emergencies, the rule of thumb for starting an intravenous infusion is "any port in a storm."

Once these five decisions have been made, then the actual procedure of inserting the IV can begin.

The procedure is as follows:

1. Receive the order.
2. Confirm the order and write it down.
3. Prepare the equipment and don gloves:

- Appropriate IV fluid
- Appropriate administration set
- Appropriate indwelling catheter
- Extension IV tubing
- Tourniquet
- Antibiotic swab
- 2 × 2 gauze pad
- 1-inch tape
- Antibiotic ointment
- Short arm board

4. Remove the envelope from the IV fluid.

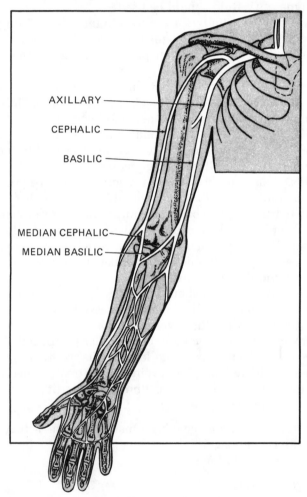

Figure 5–6   Veins of the arm.

5. Inspect the fluid, making sure that it is not discolored or containing any particulate matter; check that it contains the amount of fluid it should have. Do not administer if discolored, if particles are present, or if less than the indicated quantity of fluid is present.
6. Open and inspect the IV tubing.
7. Attach the extension tubing.
8. Close the clamp on the tubing.
9. Remove the sterile cover from the IV fluid and the administration.
10. Insert the administration set into the IV fluid.
11. Squeeze the drip chamber to fill it with fluid.
12. Bleed all of the air out of the IV tubing.
13. Hang the bag on an IV pole (or have a bystander hold it) at the appropriate height.
14. Place the tourniquet on the patient to occlude venous flow only.

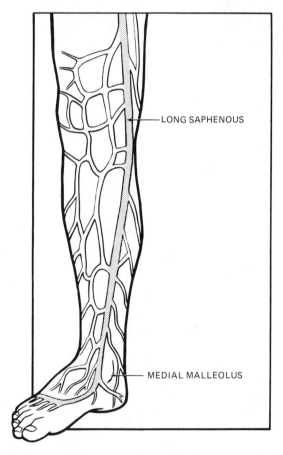

LONG SAPHENOUS

MEDIAL MALLEOLUS

Figure 5–7   Veins of the leg.

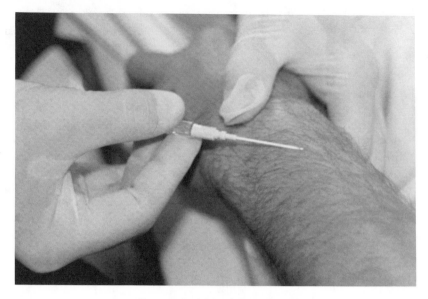

Figure 5–8 Make the puncture.

15. Select a suitable vein and palpate it (see Figures 5–6 and 5–7).
16. Prepare the site by cleansing it with an antibiotic swab.
17. Make the puncture using appropriate sterile technique, enter the vein, and advance the catheter (see Figures 5–8 and 5–9).
18. Take a blood sample.
19. Connect the IV tubing and slowly open the valve.

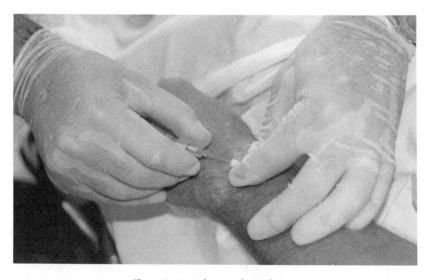

Figure 5–9 Advance the catheter.

20. Remove the tourniquet.
21. Confirm that the fluid is flowing appropriately without any evidence of infiltration.
22. Apply an antibiotic ointment over the puncture and cover with a sterile 2 × 2 gauze pad or adhesive bandage.
23. Securely tape the IV catheter and tubing down.
24. Adjust the flow rate.
25. Apply a short arm board.
26. Place the blood sample in the appropriate tubes.
27. Label the IV bag with the patient's name, date, time the IV was initiated, gauge of the catheter, and your initials.
28. Confirm the successful completion of the IV with medical control.
29. Monitor the patient for the desired effects and any undesired ones as well.

COLLECTION OF BLOOD SAMPLES FOR LABORATORY ANALYSIS

It is becoming commonplace for prehospital personnel to obtain blood samples in the field for later laboratory analysis. There are several advantages to this. It will provide the emergency department physician with information about the patient before medical intervention. This is especially true in cases of suspected hypoglycemia when 50% dextrose is administered. In situations in which a patient may be trapped, or transport to the hospital is otherwise delayed, blood samples can be taken to the hospital before the patient so that blood can be typed and cross-matched, and ready when the patient eventually arrives in the emergency department. Any time a prehospital intervention might affect the subsequent care of the patient (for example, administering Dextran that may inhibit blood typing), always draw a blood sample according to local protocol.

Most commonly, blood samples are taken when an IV is started. Always follow universal precautions when caring for a patient, and especially when handling a blood sample. Gloves and goggles should be worn. After placing the IV catheter, and before connecting the IV line, a 10-milliliter syringe can be attached to the catheter and blood gently withdrawn from the vein. The syringe can be removed and the IV line connected. It is important to withdraw the blood from the syringe slowly. Withdrawing it rapidly can damage the blood cells causing them to rupture and leak their contents. This can erroneously alter the blood chemistries rendering the sample useless.

Once blood is withdrawn from a patient it is usually placed into evacuated blood collection tubes (Vacutainer®). These tubes have a vacuum that allows the tube to fill with a predetermined amount of blood. Most tubes contain a chemical to keep the blood from clotting. Each tube has a different color rubber top depending on its use and contents. The type of tube you may be asked to draw may vary from region to region. After you have withdrawn the blood as described earlier, place an 18-gauge needle on the syringe. Insert the needle into the rubber top and allow the tube to fill with blood. Do not attempt to overfill the tube or press on the plunger of the syringe. Allow the vacuum to fill the vial.

After you have filled the vials, invert them several times to mix the blood and the anticoagulant. Immediately write the patient's name, date, time drawn, your name, and incident number (if any) on the vial. Give the tubes to the appropriate emergency department personnel on arrival. Document on the patient report form the time the blood was drawn and who you gave it to.

SUMMARY

As with the skills of medication administration, the insertion of an IV requires vigorous mannikin, classroom, and clinical training. This can only be accomplished under the supervision of a qualified instructor.

6

DRUGS USED IN TREATMENT OF CARDIOVASCULAR EMERGENCIES

INTRODUCTION

Most emergency drugs are used in the treatment of cardiac emergencies. These drugs, by the nature of their actions, may be accompanied by many side effects.

Some general classifications follow for our discussion of the emergency cardiovascular drugs:

Oxygen

- Oxygen

Sympathomimetics

- Epinephrine
- Norepinephrine (Levophed®)
- Isoproterenol (Isuprel®)
- Dopamine (Intropin®)
- Dobutamine (Dobutrex®)
- Metaraminol (Aramine®)
- Amrinone (Inocor®)

Sympathetic Blockers

- Propranolol (Inderal®)
- Metoprolol (Lopressor®)
- Labetalol (Normodyne®, Trandate®)
- Esmolol (Brevibloc®)

Antiarrhythmics

- Lidocaine (Xylocaine®)
- Bretylium tosylate (Bretylol®)
- Procainamide (Pronestyl®)
- Verapamil (Calan®, Isoptin®)
- Phenytoin (Dilantin®)
- Edrophonium chloride (Tensilon®)
- Adenosine (Adenocard®)

Parasympatholytics

- Atropine sulfate

Cardiac Glycosides

- Digoxin (Lanoxin®)

Alkalinizing Agents

- Sodium bicarbonate

Analgesics

- Morphine sulfate
- Meperidine (Demerol®)
- Nitrous oxide (Nitronox®)
- Nalbuphine (Nubain®)
- Butorphanol tartrate (Stadol®)

Diuretics

- Furosemide (Lasix®)
- Bumetanide (Bumex®)

Antianginal Agents

- Nitroglycerin (Nitrostat®)
- Nitroglycerin paste (Nitropaste®)
- Nitroglycerin spray (Nitrolingual Spray®)

Antihypertensives

- Nifedipine (Procardia®)
- Sodium nitroprusside (Nipride®)
- Hydralazine (Apresoline®)
- Diazoxide (Hyperstat®)

Other Cardiovascular Drugs

- Calcium chloride

OXYGEN

Oxygen is one of the most important emergency drugs and is required by the body to facilitate the breakdown of glucose into a usable energy form. Without oxygen the breakdown of glucose is ineffective and incomplete. This breakdown without oxygen is termed **anerobic metabolism**. Anerobic metabolism yields lactic acid, a strong acid, as its end product. This acid, in conjunction with an increased carbon dioxide level, leads to systemic acidosis.

Oxygen is an odorless, tasteless, colorless gas that vigorously supports combustion. It is present in room air at a concentration of approximately 21%. This concentration is adequate for our daily activities. In injury and illness, however, the body needs increased levels of oxygen to maintain homeostasis.

Oxygen

Description

Oxygen is an odorless, tasteless, colorless gas necessary for life. It enters the body through the respiratory system and is transported to the cells by hemoglobin, found in the red cells. Its onset of action following administration is immediate.

Indication

- Oxygen is indicated whenever hypoxia is suspected or possible. This includes all forms of trauma, medical emergencies, chest pain that may be due to cardiac ischemia, any respiratory difficulty, during labor and delivery, and in any critical patient.

Contraindications

There are no contraindications to oxygen. NEVER DEPRIVE THE HY-POXIC PATIENT OF OXYGEN FOR FEAR OF RESPIRATORY DEPRES-SION.

Precautions

Oxygen should be used cautiously in patients with chronic obstructive pulmonary disease. Respirations in these patients are often regulated by the level of oxygen in the blood (hypoxic drive), instead of carbon dioxide, and they may suffer respiratory depression if high concentrations of oxygen are delivered.

The administration of high concentrations of oxygen to neonates for a prolonged period of time can damage the infant's eyes (retrolental fibroplasia). Although this is rarely a problem in prehospital care, it is a consideration in long distance and prolonged transport.

Oxygen delivered at a flow rate of 6 liters per minute or greater should be humidified to prevent drying of the mucus membranes of the upper respiratory system.

Dosage

Cardiac arrest and other critical patients—100%
Chronic obstructive pulmonary disease—24–35% (Increase as needed)

Oxygen Delivery Device	Flow Rate (L/min)	Percentage Delivered (%)
Nasal cannula	1–6	24–44
Simple face mask	8–10	40–60
Venturi mask	4–12	24–50
Partial rebreathing mask	6–10	35–60
Nonrebreathing mask	6–10	60–95
Bas-Valve-Mask with reservoir bag	10–15	40–90
Demand valve	10–15	100

How Supplied

Oxygen is supplied in pressurized cylinders of varying size. The more common sizes include the following:

Cylinder Name	Volume (Liters)
D	400
E	660
M	3000

SYMPATHOMIMETICS

The term **sympathomimetic** means to mimic the actions of the sympathetic nervous system. Drugs in this group do exactly that. They will either act directly on receptors of the sympathetic nervous system or will act indirectly by stimulating the release of endogenous catecholamines. **Catecholamine** is the name used to describe several drugs that are chemically similar. These drugs are epinephrine, norepinephrine (Levophed®), dopamine (Intropin®), isoproterenol (Isuprel®), and dobutamine (Dobutrex®). All of these agents, except isoproteranol and dobutamine, can be found naturally in the body. Isoproterenol and dobutamine are synthetic catecholamines. To understand and appreciate the actions and roles of the sympathomimetics fully, it is essential to first review the sympathetic nervous system.

Sympathetic Nervous System

The sympathetic nervous system is sometimes called the "fight or flight" system. It is this part of the nervous system that prepares the body to deal with various stresses, whether real or imagined. Sometimes it is referred to as the **adrenergic system**. Both it, and the other aspect of the autonomic nervous system, the parasympathetic, functionally oppose each other to maintain homeostasis. The parasympathetic system is sometimes called the **cholinergic** system.

As indicated by Table 6–1, the sympathetic nervous system tends to stimulate those organs needed to deal with stressful situations. It also tends to inhibit the use of organs not needed, like the digestive tract.

The sympathetic nervous system uses the hormone norepinephrine to transmit impulses from the nerve to the effector cell. Chemicals that propagate the nervous impulse, like norepinephrine, are called **neurotransmitters**. In emergency situations the norepinephrine released by the nerve endings may be augmented with epinephrine and norepinephrine secreted from the adrenal medulla. Like the adrenergic nerves, the adrenal medulla secretes norepinephrine. About 20 percent of the catecholamines secreted by the adrenals are in the form of norepinephrine. The remaining 80 percent are in the form of epinephrine (adrenalin).

When released, norepinephrine will act on specialized receptor chemicals. These **receptors** are located at various points throughout the body. Once stimulated by the appropriate catecholamine, they will cause a response in the organ(s) they control. There are two types of receptors, the **adrenergic receptors** and the **dopaminergic receptors**. The adrenergic receptors are further divided into four different types. These four types of receptors are designated **alpha 1** (α_1), **alpha 2** (α_2), **beta 1** (β_1) and **beta 2** (β_2). The α_1 receptors cause peripheral vasoconstriction and occasionally

TABLE 6-1 Comparison of Sympathetic and Parasympathetic Actions

Organ	Sympathetic Stimulation	Parasympathetic Stimulation
Heart	Increased rate	Decreased rate
	Increased contractile force	Decreased contractile force
Lungs	Bronchodilatation	Bronchoconstriction
Kidney	Decreased output	No change
Systemic Blood Vessels		
Abdominal	Constricted	None
Muscle	Constricted (α)	None
	Dilated (β)	None
Skin	Constricted	None
Liver	Glucose release	Slight glycogen synthesis
Blood Glucose	Increased	None
Pupils	Dilated	Constricted
Sweat Glands	Copious sweating	None
Basal Metabolism	Increased up to 100%	None
Skeletal Muscle	Increased strength	None

mild bronchoconstriction. The α_2 receptors, when stimulated, inhibit the release of norepinephrine. This effect is antagonistic to the actions of α receptors and, over time, can cause peripheral vasodilation. The β_1 receptors, once stimulated, will cause an increase in cardiac rate, cardiac force, and an increase in cardiac automaticity and conduction. The β_2 receptors will cause vasodilation and bronchodilation. Dopaminergic receptors, though not totally understood, are believed to cause dilatation of the renal, coronary, and cerebral arteries.

Catecholamines

Certain drugs will stimulate certain receptors to one degree or another. Norepinephrine, for example, has an effect on both α and β receptors. However, its effects on α receptors is considerably stronger than on the β receptors. Because of this, norepinephrine is primarily regarded as an α-receptor–stimulating agent. Epinephrine, like norepinephrine, acts on both α and β receptors. However, unlike norepinephrine, epinephrine has a much greater effect on β receptors and is considered a β-receptor–stimulating agent. Isoproterenol, the synthetic catecholamine occasionally used in emergency medicine, acts entirely on β receptors with no α effects noted. Dopamine acts on both α and β receptors depending on the dosage. In addition to this, when used in certain doses, it acts on the dopaminergic receptors. This dopaminergic effect is quite useful because it tends to keep blood flowing to the renal arteries, even in emergency situations. One of the long-term major complications of severe medical emergencies, like cardiac arrest, is renal failure. Using agents like dopamine, which will maintain renal perfusion, will help in the long-term survival of the patient.

Drugs that cause an increase in the cardiac rate are called positive **chronotropic** agents. Drugs that cause an increase in cardiac force are referred to as positive **inotropic** agents.

The primary use of the sympathomimetics in emergency medicine is to increase the blood pressure in cardiogenic shock. These drugs raise the blood pressure by one of two different methods. Drugs that stimulate α receptors elevate blood pressure merely by peripheral vasoconstriction. Vasoconstriction reduces the size of the vascular pool, thus increasing the blood pressure. Drugs that act on β receptors elevate blood pressure by causing an increase in the cardiac output. Cardiac output can be defined as follows:

$$\text{Cardiac Output} = \text{Stroke Volume} \times \text{Heart Rate}$$

Thus:

$$\text{Blood Pressure} = \text{Cardiac Output} \times \text{Peripheral Resistance}$$

The β-receptor–stimulating drugs, like epinephrine and dopamine, cause both an increase in heart rate (positive chronotropic) and stroke volume (positive inotropic). The different receptor effects are summarized in Table 6–2. Table 6–3 lists many of the sympathomimetic drugs used in emergency care including their adrenergic effects and arrhythmia potential.

Epinephrine 1:10,000

Description

Epinephrine is a potent β stimulant. The 1:10,000 dilution, frequently used in the treatment of cardiac emergencies, contains 1 milligram of epinephrine in 10 milliliters of isotonic sodium chloride. When admin-

TABLE 6–2 Comparison of Effects of α and β Adrenergic Receptor Activity on Selected Organs

Organ	α-Adrenergic Receptors	β-Adrenergic Receptors
Heart	No cardiac effect	Increased heart rate (β_1) Increased contractile force (β_1) Increased automaticity (β_1)
Systemic Blood Vessels	Vasoconstriction	Vasodilatation (β_2)
Lungs	Mild bronchoconstriction	Bronchodilatation (β_2)

TABLE 6–3   Listing of Sympathomimetic Drugs with
Adrenergic Actions

Drug	Adrenergic Effects		Arrhythmia Potential
	α	β	
Epinephrine			
Low dose	+	+ +	+ + +
High dose	+ +	+ + +	+ + +
Norepinephrine			
Low dose	+ +	+	+ +
High dose	+ + +	+ +	+ +
Dopamine			
Low dose	+	+	+ +
High dose	+ + +	+ +	+ +
Isoproterenol	0	+ + +	+ + +
Dobutamine	0	+ + +	+
Amrinone	0	0	+

istered it has an effect on both α- and β-adrenergic receptors. However, its effect on β receptors is more profound. In emergency medicine, it is used to convert fine ventricular fibrillation to coarse ventricular fibrillation. This change significantly increases the chances of successful electrical defibrillation. In asystole, it is used to initiate electrical activity in the myocardium. Once initiated, electrical defibrillation may be attempted.

Because of its strong inotropic and chronotropic properties, epinephrine increases myocardial oxygen demand. When administering epinephrine in the emergency setting, these effects should be kept in mind. Like most of the other drugs used in emergency medicine, epinephrine is only effective when the myocardium is adequately oxygenated.

Epinephrine effects usually appear within 90 seconds of administration, and they are usually of short duration. Therefore, it must be administered every 5 minutes to maintain therapeutic levels.

Indications (Cardiovascular)

- Cardiac arrest

Contraindications

Epinephrine 1:10,000 is contraindicated in patients who do not require extensive cardiopulmonary resuscitative efforts. With asthma, the 1:1000 dilution is administered subcutaneously.

Precautions

Epinephrine, like all catecholamines, should be protected from light. It can be deactivated by alkaline solutions such as sodium bicarbonate. Because of this, it is essential that the IV line is adequately flushed between the administration of epinephrine and sodium bicarbonate.

Dosage

Epinephrine is administered in doses of 0.5 to 1.0 milligram. The dose should be repeated every 5 minutes until the patient is resuscitated or until resuscitation efforts have been terminated. Higher dosages may be recommended in the future.

Routes

The most common route of administration used in emergency medicine is IV. When an IV line cannot be established, however, the drug may be given endotracheally.

How Supplied

Epinephrine 1:10,000 comes in prefilled syringes containing 1 milligram of the drug in 10 milliliters of solvent.

Norepinephrine (Levophed®)

Description

Norepinephrine acts predominantly on α receptors. Thus, it is a potent peripheral vasoconstrictor. This vasoconstriction serves to increase blood pressure in cardiogenic shock and other hypotensive emergencies. Because norepinephrine also tends to constrict the renal and mesenteric blood vessels, it has fallen into relative disuse. Dopamine, which maintains renal and mesenteric perfusion, is preferred.

Indications

- Hypotension refractory to other sympathomimetics
- Neurogenic shock

Contraindications

Norepinephrine should not be given to patients who are hypotensive from hypovolemia.

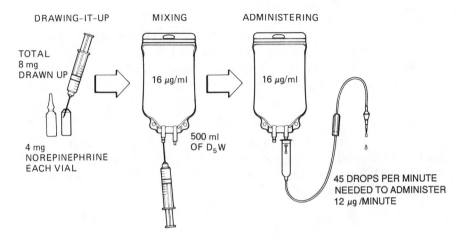

DRAWING-IT-UP   MIXING   ADMINISTERING

TOTAL
8 mg
DRAWN UP

16 µg/ml   16 µg/ml

4 mg
NOREPINEPHRINE
EACH VIAL

500 ml
OF D₅W

45 DROPS PER MINUTE
NEEDED TO ADMINISTER
12 µg /MINUTE

Figure 6–1   Preparation of norepinephrine infusion.

Precautions

Because of the powerful effects of norepinephrine, it is essential to measure the blood pressure every 5 to 10 minutes to prevent dangerously high blood pressures. Norepinephrine should be given through the largest vein readily available because it may cause local tissue necrosis. Norepinephrine can be deactivated by alkaline solutions such as sodium bicarbonate.

Dosage

The current dosage recommended by the American Heart Association for norepinephrine is 2 to 12 micrograms per minute. Higher doses may be required to maintain adequate blood pressure. The best dilution is attained by placing 8 milligrams in 500 milliliters of D_5W. This will give a concentration of 16 micrograms per milliliter. The same concentration can be attained by placing 4 milligrams in 250 milliliters of D_5W (see Figure 6–1).

Routes

Because of its potency, norepinephrine is given only in extremely diluted IV infusions. To control its administration, it should be "piggybacked" into an already established line of D_5W.

How Supplied

Norepinephrine is supplied in 4-milliliter ampules containing 4 milligrams of the drug.

Isoproterenol (Isuprel®)

Description

Isoproterenol is a potent, synthetic catecholamine that acts exclusively on β receptors. Because it has no α-receptor–stimulating capabilities, its actions are primarily on the heart and lungs. In cardiac emergencies it is used to increase heart rate in bradycardias that are refractory to atropine. Moreover, it causes an increase in cardiac output owing to its positive inotropic and chronotropic actions. It is important to be careful when administering isoproterenol. Like epinephrine, it significantly increases myocardial oxygen demand. The increase in myocardial oxygen uptake may increase myocardial infarction size. In patients who have not suffered a myocardial infarction, isoproterenol may cause myocardial ischemia. The emergency physician must weigh the benefits of isoproterenol against its risks when ordering the drug. External pacing, if available, should be used instead of isoproterenol.

Indications

- Bradycardias refractory to atropine
- Bradycardias resulting from high-degree heart blocks (that is, second-degree Mobitz II and third-degree blocks)

Contraindications

Isoproterenol is not used to increase blood pressure in cardiogenic shock. It should only be used in shock owing to bradycardias. Other sympathomimetics, like dopamine and norepinephrine, should be used in cases of cardiogenic shock.

Precautions

When administering isoproterenol, the patient must be monitored for signs of ventricular irritability. These may take the form of premature ventricular contractions, ventricular tachycardia, or even ventricular fibrillation. Lidocaine should be readily available whenever administering isoproterenol.

Because isoproterenol causes significant increases in myocardial oxygen demand, it should be avoided in cases of acute myocardial infarction whenever possible.

Isoproterenol can be deactivated by alkaline solutions such as sodium bicarbonate.

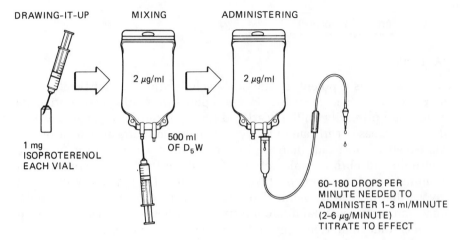

Figure 6–2   Preparation of isoproterenol infusion.

Dosage

One milligram of isoproterenol should be diluted in 500 milliliters of D_5W. This will give a concentration of 2 micrograms per milliliter. It should be titrated until the desired heart rate is attained or until signs of ventricular irritability, such as premature ventricular contractions, occur. The recommended infusion rate is 2 to 10 micrograms per minute (see Figure 6–2).

Route

Because of its potency, isoproterenol should only be given by IV infusion. An established line of D_5W, into which the isoproterenol is piggybacked, should be maintained.

How Supplied

Isoproterenol is supplied in ampules containing 1 milligram in either 1 milliliter or 5 milliliters of solvent. Prefilled syringes, designed especially for IV infusion preparation, are available.

Dopamine (Intropin®)

Description

Dopamine is one of the most commonly used agents in the treatment of hypotension associated with cardiogenic shock. It is chemically related to both epinephrine and norepinephrine. Dopamine acts primarily on β_1

receptors exerting a positive inotropic effect on the heart. The drug does not cause an increase in myocardial oxygen demand as much as isoproterenol and does not have the same powerful chronotropic effects. Unlike norepinephrine, when used in therapeutic dosages, dopamine maintains renal and mesenteric blood flow. For these reasons, dopamine is the most commonly used vasopressor. Dopamine will usually increase the systolic blood pressure and the pulse pressure (the difference between the systolic and diastolic blood pressures), but as a rule, there is usually less effect on the diastolic pressure.

Indications

- Cardiogenic shock
- Hypotension (systolic pressure less than 90 millimeters of mercury) not resulting from hypovolemia.

Contraindications

Dopamine should not be used as the sole agent in the management of hypovolemic shock unless fluid resuscitation is well under way. Dopamine should not be used in patients with pheochromocytoma.

Precautions

Dopamine should not be administered in the presence of tachyarrhythmias or ventricular fibrillation. Like all of the vasopressors, it can be deactivated by alkaline solutions, such as sodium bicarbonate. If the patient is taking monoamine oxidase inhibitors, the dose should then be reduced.

Dosage

The standard method of preparing a dopamine infusion is to place 800 milligrams in 500 milliliters of D$_5$W. This dilution can be attained by adding 400 milligrams to 250 milliliters of D$_5$W. This gives a concentration of 1600 micrograms per milliliter. The effects of dopamine are dose dependent. Table 6–4 illustrates effects based on common dosages.

The initial infusion rate is from 2 to 5 micrograms per kilogram per minute. This may be increased until blood pressure improves (see Figure 6–3).

Routes

Dopamine is administered only by IV infusion, which should be piggybacked into an already established infusion of D$_5$W.

TABLE 6–4 Dopamine Hydrochloride (Intropin®) Dosage Phenomena

Effects of Intropin at Three Dose Ranges	2–5 mcg/kg/min	5–20 mcg/kg/min	More Than 20 mcg/kg/min
Cardiac Output	No change	Increase	Increase
Stroke Volume	No change	Increase	Increase
Heart Rate	No change	There is an initial increase followed by a decrease toward normal rates as infusion continues	
Myocardial Contractility	No change	Increase	Increase
Potential for Excessive Myocardial Oxygen Demands	Low[a]	Low[a]	Data unavailable
	Coronary blood flow increased	Coronary blood flow increased	
Potential for Tachyarrhythmias	Low[a]	Low[a]	Moderate
Total Systemic Vascular Resistance	Slight decrease to no change	No change to slight increase	Increase
Renal Blood Flow	Increase	Increase	Decrease[b]
Urine Output	Increase	Increase	Decrease[b]

[a]Low but needs monitoring.
[b]Relative to peak values achieved at lower dosages.
©1981 American Critical Care Division of American Hospital Supply Corporation
(*Courtesy of American Critical Care, Division of American Hospital Supply Corporation, McGaw Park, Illinois, 1983*).

TABLE 6–5 Dopamine Hydrochloride (Intropin®) Dosage Chart

For a concentration of 1600 µg dopamine hydrochloride/ml (800 mg Intropin per 500 ml—or—400 mg Intropin per 250 ml)

Flow Rate in Drops[a] per Minute

Dosage = mcg Dopamine hydrochloride/kg/min

Body Wt lbs	Body Wt kgs	5	10	15	20	25	30	35	40	45	50	55	60	70	80	90	100
242	110	3.8	7.6	11	15	19	23	27	31	34	38	42	46	53	61	69	76
231	105	3.6	7.3	11	15	18	22	25	29	33	36	40	44	51	58	65	73
220	100	3.5	6.9	10	14	17	21	24	28	31	35	38	41	48	55	62	69
209	95	3.3	6.6	9.8	13	16	20	23	26	30	33	36	39	46	53	59	66
198	90	3.1	6.2	9.3	12	16	19	22	25	28	31	34	37	44	50	56	62
187	85	2.9	5.9	8.8	12	15	18	21	23	26	29	32	35	41	47	53	59
176	80	2.8	5.5	8.3	11	14	17	19	22	25	28	30	33	39	44	50	55
165	75	2.6	5.2	7.8	10	13	16	18	21	23	26	28	31	36	41	47	52
154	70	2.4	4.8	7.3	9.7	12	15	17	19	22	24	27	29	34	39	44	48
143	65	2.25	4.5	6.7	9.0	11	13	16	18	20	22	25	27	31	36	40	45
132	60	2.1	4.1	6.2	8.3	10	12	15	17	19	21	23	25	29	33	37	41
121	55	1.9	3.8	5.7	7.6	9.5	11	13	15	17	19	21	23	27	30	34	38
110	50	1.7	3.5	5.2	6.9	8.6	10	12	14	16	17	19	21	24	28	31	35
99	45	1.55	3.1	4.7	6.2	7.8	9.3	11	12	14	16	17	19	22	25	28	31
88	40	1.4	2.8	4.1	5.5	6.9	8.3	9.7	11	12	14	15	17	19	22	25	28
77	35	1.2	2.4	3.6	4.9	6.0	7.3	8.5	9.7	11	12	13	15	17	19	22	24

[a]Based on a microdrip calibration of 60 drops equal to 1.0 milliliter.

Note: All dosages of 10 µg/kg/min and greater have been rounded off to the nearest µg/kg/min.

(Courtesy of American Critical Care, Division of American Hospital Supply Corporation, McGaw Park, Illinois, 1983.)

87

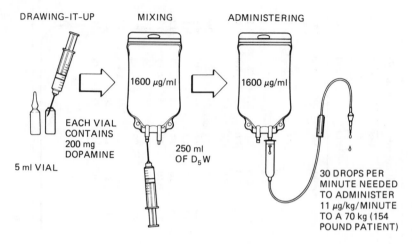

DRAWING-IT-UP   MIXING   ADMINISTERING

EACH VIAL CONTAINS 200 mg DOPAMINE

5 ml VIAL

1600 μg/ml

250 ml OF D₅W

1600 μg/ml

30 DROPS PER MINUTE NEEDED TO ADMINISTER 11 μg/kg/MINUTE TO A 70 kg (154 POUND PATIENT)

Figure 6–3   Preparation of dopamine infusion.

How Supplied

Dopamine comes in prefilled syringes and ampules. The standard preparation is 200 milligrams in 5 milliliters of solvent; 400 milligram preparations in 5 milliliters of solvent are also available.

Dobutamine (Dobutrex®)

Description

Dobutamine, like isoproterenol, is a synthetic catecholamine. It acts primarily on β receptors but is less of a β agonist than isoproterenol. Dobutamine increases the force of the systolic contraction (positive inotropic effect) with little chronotropic activity. For these reasons, it is useful in the management of congestive heart failure when an increase in heart rate is not desired.

Indication

- Short-term management of congestive heart failure when an increased cardiac output, without an increase in cardiac rate, is desired.

Contraindications

Dobutamine should not be used as the sole agent in hypovolemic shock unless fluid resuscitation is well under way. To increase cardiac output in severe emergencies, like cardiogenic shock, dopamine is the preferred agent.

Precautions

Tachycardia and an increase in the systolic blood pressure are common following the administration of dobutamine. Increases in heart rate of more than 10 percent may induce or exacerbate myocardial ischemia. Premature ventricular contractions (PVCs) can occur in conjunction with dobutamine administration. Lidocaine should be readily available. As with any sympathomimetic, blood pressure should be monitored.

Dosage

The desired dosage range for dobutamine is between 2.5 and 20 micrograms per kilogram per minute. Dobutamine should be administered according to the patient's response (see Figure 6–4).

Route

Dobutamine should be diluted in either 500 milliliters or 1 liter of D_5W and administered via IV infusion.

How Supplied

Dobutamine is supplied in 20-milliliter ampules containing 250 milligrams of the drug; 250 milligrams is usually placed in 500 milliliters of solvent to give a concentration of 0.5 milligram (500 micrograms) per milliliter.

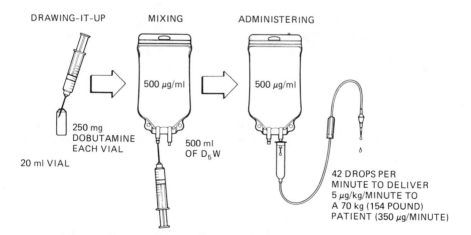

DRAWING-IT-UP   MIXING   ADMINISTERING

250 mg DOBUTAMINE EACH VIAL

20 ml VIAL

500 µg/ml

500 µg/ml

500 ml OF D_5W

42 DROPS PER MINUTE TO DELIVER 5 µg/kg/MINUTE TO A 70 kg (154 POUND) PATIENT (350 µg/MINUTE)

Figure 6–4   Preparation of dobutamine infusion.

Metaraminol (Aramine®)

Description

Although metaraminol is not a catecholamine, it is used in the treatment of hypotensive states. It is both an α and β agonist. Its vasopressor properties are primarily derived from its action on endogenous catecholamines. In recent years, metaraminol has fallen into disuse, with dopamine being the preferred agent.

Indication

- Hypotension resulting from cardiogenic shock is the primary indication.

Contraindications

Metaraminol should not be used in hypovolemia unless fluid resuscitation is well under way.

Precautions

Rapid administration can cause hypertension. Ventricular ectopic activity, especially PVCs, has been known to occur with the administration of metaraminol. Lidocaine should be readily available. Caution should be used in digitalized patients.

Dosage

Two hundred milligrams of metaraminol should be placed into 500 milligrams of D_5W. This will give a dilution of 0.4 milligrams per milliliter. The infusion rate should be titrated according to the blood pressure response.

Route

Metaraminol should be given by IV infusion only. An infusion of D_5W should already be established into which the metaraminol should be piggybacked.

How Supplied

Metaraminol comes in a concentration of 10 milligrams per milliliter. Ampules contain either 1 or 10 milliliters. Thus, each ampule will contain 10 and 100 milligrams, respectively.

Amrinone (Inocor®)

Description

Amrinone, like the other medications previously presented, increases cardiac output promptly following intravenous administration. It is a positive inotrope and does possess some vasodilatory properties. Unlike the other medications, however, it does not stimulate either α or β-adrenergic receptors. The exact mechanism by which amrinone increases blood pressure is not well understood. It does not increase cardiac output in the same manner as the digitalis preparations. Clinically, amrinone resembles dobutamine in its effects. Because amrinone does not stimulate β-adrenergic receptors, it may be effective in cases of congestive heart failure that do not respond to dobutamine or one of the other inotropic agents.

Indication

- Short-term management of congestive heart failure not associated with myocardial infarction.

Contraindications

Amrinone should not be administered to patients with a known hypersensitivity to the drug or to the bisulfite class of chemicals.

Precautions

Amrinone should not be used in cases of congestive heart failure occurring immediately after myocardial infarction. Like dobutamine, amrinone may increase myocardial ischemia. As with the other inotropic agents, the blood pressure, pulse, and electrocardiogram (EKG) should be constantly monitored.

Amrinone should not be diluted in solutions containing dextrose (that is, D_5W). Amrinone should be diluted with 0.9% sodium chloride (normal saline) or 0.45% sodium chloride ($\frac{1}{2}$ normal saline).

Furosemide (Lasix) should not be administered into an intravenous line delivering amrinone. A chemical reaction occurs between these two drugs resulting in the formation of a precipitate in the intravenous line.

Dosage

Therapy should be initiated with an IV bolus of 0.75 milligrams per kilogram given slowly during a 2- to 3-minute interval (see Figure 6–5).

This should be followed by a maintenance infusion of 2 to 20 micrograms per kilogram per minute. This infusion can be prepared by placing

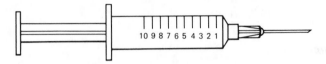

Figure 6–5   Loading bolus of amrinone.

one ampule (100 milligrams) in 500 milliliters of normal saline solution. This will give a concentration of 0.2 milligram per milliliter (200 micrograms per milliliter) (see Figure 6–6).

An additional bolus of 0.75 milligram per kilogram given slowly over 2 to 3 minutes can be given 30 minutes later if required.

The overall rate of amrinone administration must be carefully adjusted and based on the patient's clinical response.

Route

Amrinone should only be administered by the IV route, either as a bolus or infusion, as described earlier.

How Supplied

Amrinone is supplied in 20-milliliter ampules containing 5 milligrams per milliliter.

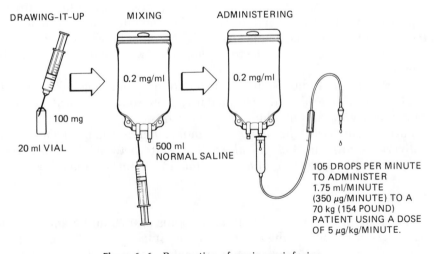

Figure 6–6   Preparation of amrinone infusion.

SYMPATHETIC BLOCKERS

Sympathetic blockers are a unique class of drugs that antagonize adrenergic receptor sites. Certain drugs will block only α receptors, whereas others block only β receptors. Some of the β blockers are so selective that they block only β_1 or β_2 receptors. The drugs that block the β receptors are receiving the most use. They are useful in the treatment of hypertension, cardiac arrhythmias, and angina pectoris. The most popular sympathetic blocker is propranolol (Inderal®), a nonselective beta blocker that is both a β_1 and β_2 antagonist. Although used selectively in emergency medicine, propranolol does play a role in the treatment of certain cardiac arrhythmias.

It is thought that some ventricular arrhythmias, such as ventricular tachycardia and recurrent ventricular fibrillation, can be caused by excessive β stimulation.

Administration of propranolol may inhibit these arrhythmias. Propranolol should not be used in combination with verapamil. The concomitant blocking of slow calcium channels by verapamil, and the β antagonism caused by propranolol, may result in asystole. (Verapamil will be discussed in detail on page 107).

Propranolol (Inderal®)

Description

Propranolol is a nonselective β antagonist. It is useful in treating ventricular tachycardia or recurrent ventricular fibrillation that does not respond to lidocaine. It may also be of value in the treatment of tachyarrhythmias resulting from digitalis toxicity and selected supraventricular tachycardias.

Indications

- Ventricular tachycardia refractory to lidocaine and bretylium
- Recurrent ventricular fibrillation refractory to lidocaine and bretylium
- Selected supraventricular tachyarrhythmias

Contraindications

Propranolol is contraindicated in patients with bradycardia, a history of asthma, chronic obstructive pulmonary disease (COPD), and congestive heart failure.

Precautions

Propranolol should not be administered to patients who have received verapamil. Because propranolol may decrease heart rate, atropine should be readily available. In bradycardia refractory to atropine, isoproterenol should be tried.

Dosage

Propranolol may produce significant, even life-threatening, side effects. When administered intravenously, care must be taken to dilute 1 milligram in 10 milliliters of D_5W. The standard dosage is 1 to 3 milligrams, diluted in 10 to 30 milliliters of D_5W. Propranolol should be administered *slowly*. Throughout administration, careful blood pressure monitoring is required. It, like all drugs acting on the heart, should only be administered on patients who are on cardiac monitors. The dosage may be repeated, again under careful monitoring, until a maximum of 3 to 5 milligrams has been administered.

Route

Propranolol is administered intravenously in the treatment of life-threatening tachyarrhythmias.

How Supplied

The standard preparation of propranolol comes in 1 milliliter vials containing 1 milligram of the drug.

Metoprolol (Lopressor®)

Description

Metoprolol is a β antagonist that blocks both β_1 and β_2 adrenergic receptors. Unlike propranolol, however, metoprolol is selective for β_1 adrenergic receptors, which results in a reduction in heart rate, systolic blood pressure, and cardiac output following administration. In addition, metoprolol appears to inhibit tachycardia, especially in the period following an acute myocardial infarction. Because of these effects, metoprolol is thought to be protective of the heart and is used in selected patients who have suffered an acute myocardial infarction to reduce potential complications. Metoprolol has proved effective in reducing the incidence of ventricular fibrillation and chest pain in these patients, thus reducing overall patient mortality in the postmyocardial infarction period.

Indication

- Patients with suspected or definite acute myocardial infarction who are hemodynamically stable.

Contraindications

Metoprolol is contraindicated in any patient with a heart rate of less than 45 beats per minute, a systolic blood pressure less than 100 millimeters of mercury, or congestive heart failure. In addition, metoprolol is contraindicated in patients with first-degree heart block with a PR interval greater than 0.24 second, a second-degree heart block (either Mobitz I or Mobitz II), or third-degree block. It is also contraindicated in any patient showing either early or late signs of shock.

Metoprolol should not be administered to any patient with a history of asthma or bronchospastic disease in the prehospital setting.

Precautions

The blood pressure, pulse rate, EKG, and respiratory status should be continuously monitored during metoprolol therapy. Prehospital personnel should be alert for signs and symptoms of congestive heart failure, bradycardia, shock, heart block, or bronchospasm when administering metoprolol. The presence of any of these signs or symptoms is an indication for discontinuing the medication.

Dosage

When administered following an acute myocardial infarction, an initial bolus of 5 milligrams metoprolol should be given by slow IV injection. If the vital signs remain stable, a second 5-milligram bolus should be given 2 minutes after the first. Finally, if the first two boluses are well tolerated, a third 5-milligram bolus should be administered 2 minutes after the second bolus. The total dose should not exceed 15 milligrams. As mentioned previously, the vital signs and EKG should be constantly monitored.

Route

Metoprolol should only be administered by slow IV infusion in the manner described earlier.

How Supplied

Metoprolol (Lopressor®) is supplied in ampules and prefilled syringes containing 5 milligrams of the drug in 5 milliliters of solvent.

Labetalol (Trandate®, Normodyne®)

Description

Labetalol differs considerably in its action from the β blockers previously presented. Like propranolol, labetalol is a nonselective β adrenergic antagonist showing no preference for either β_1 or β_2 receptors. However, unlike the other β blockers, labetalol also blocks α_1 adrenergic receptors. Blockage of α_1 receptors inhibits peripheral vasoconstriction, thus causing peripheral vasodilitation. Because of these properties labetalol is a potent agent for lowering blood pressure in cases of hypertensive crisis. It does this by decreasing cardiac output through its β_1 blocking properties and by causing peripheral vasodilatation through its α_1 blocking properties.

Indication

- Labetalol is indicated for the acute management of hypertensive crisis.

Contraindications

Labetalol is contraindicated in patients with bronchial asthma, congestive heart failure, heart block, bradycardia, or cardiogenic shock.

Precautions

As with all β blockers the blood pressure, pulse rate, EKG, and respiratory status should be continuously monitored. Prehospital personnel should be alert for signs and symptoms of congestive heart failure, bradycardia, shock, heart block, or bronchospasm when administering labetalol. The appearance of any of these signs or symptoms is an indication for discontinuing the drug.

Because of the effects of labetalol on α_1 receptors, postural hypotension might occur and should be anticipated. The patient should be supine at all times during drug administration.

Dosage

The following are two accepted methods of administering labetalol in the treatment of hypertensive crisis:

1. Twenty milligrams of labetalol can be administered by slow IV injection over 2 minutes. Immediately before the injection and at 5 and 10 minutes after the injection the supine blood pressure should be recorded. Additional injections of 40 milligrams can be given every 10 minutes until a desired supine blood pressure is achieved or 300 milligrams of the drug has been given (see Figure 6–7).

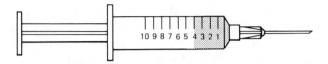

Figure 6–7   Bolus administration of labetalol.

2. Two ampules (200 milligrams) of labetalol can be added to 250 milliliters of D_5W. This gives a concentration of 0.8 milligram per milliliter. This solution should be administered at a rate of 2 milligrams per minute (2.5 milliliters per minute). The blood pressure should be continuously monitored (see Figure 6–8).

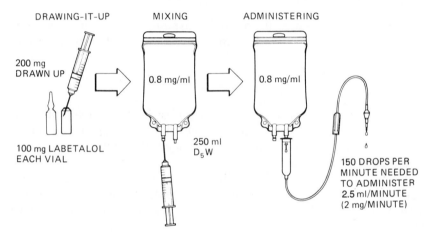

Figure 6–8   Preparation of labetalol infusion.

Route

Labetalol should be administered by slow IV injection or infusion as described earlier.

How Supplied

Labetalol (Trandate®, Normodyne®) is supplied in ampules containing 100 milligrams in 20 milliliters of solvent (5 milligrams per milliliter).

Esmolol (Brevibloc®)

Description

Esmolol (Brevibloc®) is a β_1 selective (cardioselective) β blocker with a very short half-life. Once administered, it has a very rapid onset and a short duration of action (9 minutes). Esmolol is used to slow rapid heart rates in patients with supraventricular tachycardia including atrial flutter and atrial fibrillation. Patients with extremely rapid heart rates can develop congestive heart failure or angina because the rapid heart rate may prevent adequate filling of the ventricles. The duration of action of esmolol is so brief that it should be administered by intravenous infusion.

Indication

- Supraventricular tachycardia (including atrial fibrillation and atrial flutter) accompanied by a rapid ventricular rate.

Contraindications

Esmolol should not be used in patients with sinus bradycardia, heart block greater than first degree, cardiogenic shock, and overt congestive heart failure.

Precautions

A significant number of patients receiving esmolol may experience hypotension (systolic less than 90 millimeters of mercury). Hypotension can occur at any dose but primarily is dose related. If hypotension develops, the dosage should be reduced.

Patients with congestive heart failure may have worsening of their symptoms with esmolol. Because esmolol can potentially depress cardiac contractility, it should be used with extreme caution in patients prone to congestive heart failure.

Patients with bronchospastic disease (asthma, COPD) should not receive β blockers, including esmolol, unless the medical control physician deems the benefits outweigh the risks.

Dosage

Esmolol therapy is started by administering a loading dose of 500 micrograms per kilogram per minute for 1 minute. After 1 minute this should be reduced to a maintenance dose of 50 micrograms per kilogram per minute for 4 minutes. If an adequate therapeutic effect is not seen, repeat the loading dose for 1 minute, then increase the maintenance dose to 100 micrograms per kilogram per minute. The dose can be titrated at 4-minute intervals by repeating the loading dose for 1 minute and increasing the maintenance dose by 50 micrograms per kilogram per minute at 4-minute intervals until the desired effect is obtained. The maintenance dose should not exceed 200 micrograms per kilogram per minute. In the event of an adverse reaction the dose of esmolol can be reduced or discontinued immediately (see Figure 6–9).

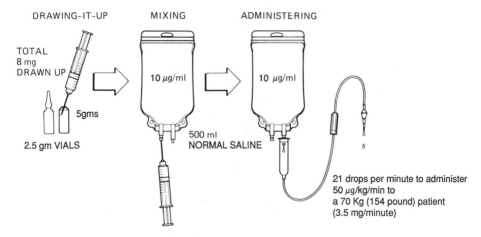

Figure 6–9   Administration of Brevibloc.

The esmolol infusion is prepared by placing two 2.5-gram ampules of esmolol in 500 milliliters of 5% dextrose, normal saline, or lactated Ringer's. An alternative method is to place one 2.5-gram ampule in 250 milliliters of fluid. Either will provide a 10-milligrams per milliliter concentration.

Route

Esmolol should be administered intravenously.

How Supplied

Esmolol is supplied in 100 milligram vials containing 100 milligrams in 10 milliliters (10 milligrams per milliliter) for loading-dose administration. It is also supplied in 2.5-gram vials for preparation of the infusion. *The 2.5-gram vials are for preparation of the infusion only, not for intravenous injection.*

ANTIARRHYTHMICS

Many different drugs are useful in the treatment and prevention of cardiac arrhythmias. Some drugs are useful in the treatment of atrial arrhythmias, whereas others are useful in the treatment of ventricular arrhythmias. As a result, it is essential to distinguish between arrhythmias of ventricular and those of an atrial origin. The common antiarrhythmic drugs are classified based on their action (see Table 6–6).

TABLE 6–6   Classification of Antiarrhythmic Agents

Class	Drugs
I	A. Procainamide (Pronestyl®) Disopyramide (Norpace®) Quinidine (Quiniglute®) B. Lidocaine (Xylocaine®) Phenytoin (Dilantin®) Mexilitine (Mexitil®) Tocainide (Tonocard®) C. Flecanide (Tambocor®) Encainide (Enkaid®)
II	Propranolol (Inderal®) Atenolol (Tenormin®) Labetolol (Trandate®, Normodyne®) Metoprolol (Lopressor®) Esmolol (Brevibloc®)
III	Bretylium (Bretylol®) Amiodarone (Cordarone®)
IV	Verapamil (Isoptin®, Calan®) Diltiazem (Cardizen®) Nefedipine (Procardia®) Nicardipine (Cardene®)

The most common antiarrhythmic drugs used in emergency medicine include the following:

Lidocaine (Xylocaine®). Lidocaine is the drug of choice in the treatment of ventricular tachycardia and malignant premature ventricular contractions.

Bretylium Tosylate (Bretylol®). Bretylium is used in the treatment of ventricular fibrillation that is refractory to lidocaine.

Verapamil (Isoptin®). Verapamil is a slow channel calcium blocker. It is a first-line drug used in the treatment of paroxysmal supraventricular tachycardia and other atrial arrhythmias.

Procainamide (Pronestyl®). Procainamide, like lidocaine, is useful in the suppression of ventricular arrhythmias. It is generally not a first-line drug, and its use is reserved for arrhythmias that do not respond to lidocaine.

Phenytoin (Dilantin®). Phenytoin is infrequently used in the emergency setting as an antiarrhythmic agent. It has proven effectiveness, however, in the management of life-threatening arrhythmias resulting from digitalis toxicity.

Edrophonium Chloride (Tensilon®). Edrophonium chloride is an anticholinesterase agent that has proven effectiveness in terminating paroxysmal supraventricular tachycardias that do not respond to vagal maneuvers. Its usage is rapidly declining with verapamil and adenosine being preferred.

Propranolol (Inderal®). Propranolol, discussed in the previous section, plays a role in the treatment of supraventricular arrhythmias. Students are encouraged to review the section on propranolol and integrate it with the drugs mentioned here.

Lidocaine (Xylocaine®)

Description

Lidocaine is probably the most frequently used antiarrhythmic agent in the treatment of life-threatening cardiac emergencies. Moreover, it has been shown to be effective in suppressing premature ventricular contractions, treating ventricular tachycardia and some cases of ventricular fibrillation, and in increasing the fibrillation threshold in acute myocardial infarction.

The most common cause of ventricular arrhythmias is acute myocardial infarction. Lidocaine suppresses ventricular ectopy in the setting of myocardial infarction and increases the ventricular fibrillation threshold. This prevents PVCs from inducing ventricular fibrillation. After acute myocardial infarction, the ventricular fibrillation threshold is often significantly reduced. Moreover, because electrical defibrillation tends to cause ventricular irritability, patients who have been successfully defibrillated should be treated with lidocaine.

Lidocaine seems to be successful in suppressing ventricular arrhythmias only when the level of the drug in the blood is between 1.5 and 6.0 micrograms per milliliter of blood. A 75-milligram to 100-milligram bolus of lidocaine will maintain adequate blood levels for only 20 minutes (see Figure 6–10). Therefore, a lidocaine bolus should be followed by a 2- to 4-milligrams per minute infusion to assure therapeutic blood levels (see Figure 6–11). It is important to distinguish patterns of premature ven-

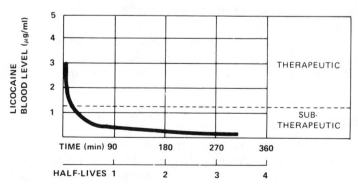

Figure 6–10 Blood levels of lidocaine following bolus without drip.

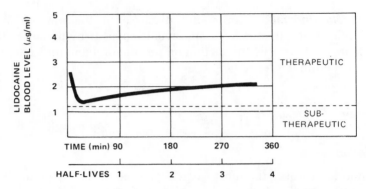

Figure 6–11   Blood levels of lidocaine following bolus with drip.

tricular contractions that are likely to lead to serious arrhythmias. Premature ventricular contractions that may lead to life-threatening arrhythmias are called **malignant premature ventricular contractions**. These include the following:

- More than six unifocal PVCs per minute
- PVCs that appear to be coming from more than one ectopic focus (for example, multifocal PVCs)
- PVCs that occur in couplets (two PVCs together without a normal QRS complex in between)
- Runs of more than two PVCs, or ventricular tachycardia
- PVCs falling in the vulnerable period of the preceding normal complex (R on T phenomena).

The aforementioned premature ventricular contractions, as well as ventricular tachycardia and ventricular fibrillation, must be treated vigorously with lidocaine.

Indications

- Malignant premature ventricular contractions
- Ventricular tachycardia
- Ventricular fibrillation (after the initial series of resuscitative procedures including electrical defibrillation)
- Prophylaxis of arrhythmias associated with acute myocardial infarction

Contraindications

Lidocaine is usually contraindicated in second-degree Mobitz II and third-degree blocks. Lidocaine slows conduction of the electrical impulse from the atria to the ventricles. Decreased ventricular rates may accompany high-grade heart block, resulting in escape beats that are premature ventricular contractions. Whenever premature ventricular contractions occur in conjunction with bradycardia (heart rate less than 60), the bradycardia should be treated first. The drug of choice is atropine sulfate, followed by external pacing or isoproterenol if atropine is not effective. If PVCs are still present after increasing the rate, lidocaine should be administered.

Precautions

Central nervous system depression may occur when the dosage exceeds 300 milligrams per hour. Symptoms of central nervous system depression include a decreased level of consciousness, irritability, confusion, muscle twitching, and, eventually, seizures. Exceedingly high doses can result in coma and death.

Dosage

The initial dose of lidocaine should be 1 milligram per kilogram unless the patient is older than 70 years of age. Additional boluses of 0.5 milligram per kilogram can be administered at 8- to 10-minute intervals until the arrhythmia is suppressed or until 3 milligrams per kilogram of the drug has been administered. After the arrhythmia has been suppressed, and the patient has adequate circulatory function, a continuous infusion should be started at 2 to 4 milligrams per minute. Continuous IV infusion should not be used in cardiac arrest. In patients older than 70 years of age the lidocaine dose should be reduced by 50% (see Figure 6–12).

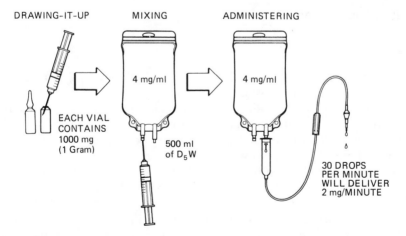

Figure 6–12   Preparation of lidocaine infusion.

Routes

Lidocaine is generally given in an IV bolus followed by an infusion. It can also be given endotracheally, however, when an IV line cannot be established. A preparation of lidocaine is also available that can be given intramuscularly for ventricular arrhythmias. This should be reserved for times when an IV line cannot be established, and the patient is not intubated.

How Supplied

Lidocaine is supplied in the following dosages:

Prefilled Syringes

- 100 milligrams in 5 milliliters of solvent
- 1- and 2-gram additive syringes

Ampules

- 100 milligrams in 5 milliliters of solvent
- 1- and 2-gram vials (in 30 milliliters of solvent)

Premixed Bags

- Premixed bags containing 1 to 2 grams in 500 milliliters of 5% dextrose.

Bretylium Tosylate (Bretylol®)

Description

Bretylium tosylate is a relatively new antiarrhythmic drug. Approved for use in 1978, bretylium tosylate has proved effective in the treatment of ventricular fibrillation and ventricular tachycardia. Its use is reserved, however, for those patients who fail to respond to lidocaine or other first-line antiarrhythmics. It has been demonstrated that bretylium increases the ventricular fibrillation threshold, much like lidocaine. It appears that bretylium raises the ventricular fibrillation threshold through postganglionic adrenergic blockade. A side effect of this blockade is bradycardia and postural hypotension, which is commonly seen within 24 hours after the administration of bretylium. Bretylium will *sometimes* convert ventricular fibrillation or ventricular tachycardia to a supraventricular rhythm. Because of this action, bretylium is sometimes referred to as a "chemical defibrillator."

Bretylium's effects are usually not evident until 5 to 10 minutes after administration, and subsequently cardiopulmonary resuscitative procedures should be continued in the interim.

Indications

- Ventricular fibrillation refractory to lidocaine
- Ventricular tachycardia refractory to lidocaine

At present, bretylium is not considered a first-line antiarrhythmic.

Contraindications

There are no contraindications to bretylium when used in the treatment of life-threatening ventricular arrhythmias.

Precautions

Postural hypotension occurs in approximately 50 percent of the patients receiving bretylium. This side effect should be anticipated, and the patient should be kept in a supine position.

Dosage

Bretylium should be administered at a dose of 5 milligrams per kilogram body weight. If the arrhythmia persists, a second dose of 10 milligrams per kilogram should be administered. The total dose should not exceed 30 milligrams per kilogram.

Routes

Because bretylium is somewhat slow in its onset, it should be administered by IV bolus.

How Supplied

Bretylium is supplied in ampules containing 500 milligrams of the drug in 10 milliliters of solvent.

Procainamide (Pronestyl®)

Description

Procainamide is still used in the treatment of ventricular arrhythmias. Because lidocaine is the drug of choice in treating ventricular arrhythmias, procainamide should be withheld until at least 225 milligrams of lidocaine have been administered and found to be unsuccessful in treating ventricular ectopy.

Indications

- Premature ventricular contractions refractory to lidocaine
- Ventricular tachycardia refractory to lidocaine

Contraindications

Procainamide should not be administered to patients with severe conduction system disturbances, especially second- and third-degree heart blocks.

Precautions

Procainamide must not be administered to patients demonstrating PVCs in conjunction with a bradycardia. The heart rate should be first increased with atropine or isoproterenol. Only after increasing the heart rate can the PVCs be treated with lidocaine or procainamide.

Hypotension is common with intravenous infusion. Constant blood pressure monitoring is essential.

Dosage

In treating PVCs or ventricular tachycardia, 100 milligrams should be administered very 5 minutes at a rate of 20 milligrams per minute. This should be discontinued if any of the following occur:

- Arrhythmia is suppressed.
- Hypotension ensues.
- QRS complex is widened by 50 percent of its original width.
- A total of 1 gram of the medication has been administered.

The maintenance infusion of procainamide is 1 to 4 milligrams per minute. The duration of procainamide's effect is shorter than lidocaine requiring a more rigorous approach.

Routes

Procainamide should be administered by slow IV bolus (20 milligrams per minute) followed by a maintenance infusion.

How Supplied

Procainamide is supplied in the following:

- 10-milliliter vials containing 1000 milligrams of the drug
- 2-milliliter vials containing 1000 milligrams of the drug (for infusion)

Verapamil (Isoptin® Calan®)

Description

Verapamil is a calcium ion antagonist and tends to slow conduction through the atrioventricular (AV) node. The advantages of this are twofold. First, verapamil will inhibit arrhythmias caused by a reentry mechanism such as supraventricular tachycardia. Second, it will decrease the rapid ventricular response seen with atrial tachyarrhythmias such as atrial flutter and fibrillation. Verapamil also reduces myocardial oxygen demand because of its negative inotropic effects and causes coronary and peripheral vasodilation.

Indication

- Paroxysmal supraventricular tachycardia (PSVT)

Contraindications

Verapamil should not be administered to any patient with severe hypotension or cardiogenic shock. In addition, verapamil should not be administered to patients with ventricular tachycardia in the prehospital setting.

Before attempting to treat a patient suffering atrial flutter or atrial fibrillation it is essential that the paramedic assure that the patient does not suffer from Wolff-Parkinson-White syndrome.

Note: Verapamil should not be administered to patients receiving intravenous β blockers.

Precautions

Verapamil can cause systemic hypotension. Because of this it is essential that the blood pressure be constantly monitored following verapamil administration.

Dosage

In the treatment of paroxysmal supraventricular tachycardia, a 3- to 5-milligram IV dose should be given initially during a 2- to 3-minute interval. A second dose of 5 to 10 milligrams can be given after 30 minutes if PSVT persists, and there has not been any adverse responses to the initial dose. The total dose of verapamil should not exceed 15 milligrams in 30 minutes.

How Supplied

Verapamil (Isoptin®) is supplied in 2-milliliter ampules containing 5 milligrams of the drug.

Phenytoin (Dilantin®)

Description

Phenytoin (Dilantin®) is used frequently in the treatment of epilepsy but also has antiarrhythmic properties. It has proved effective in the management of arrhythmias caused by digitalis toxicity or tricyclic drug overdoses. Its use in the management of status epilepticus is discussed in Chapter 9.

Indication

- Phenytoin is indicated for treatment of life-threatening arrhythmias resulting from digitalis toxicity or tricyclic antidepressant overdose. Ventricular arrhythmias in the setting of acute myocardial infarction should first be treated with lidocaine.

Contraindications

Phenytoin is contraindicated in cases of bradycardia and high-grade heart block.

Precautions

Intravenous administration of phenytoin should not exceed 50 milligrams per minute. Signs of central nervous system depression or hypotension may occur. Avoid extravasation.

Dosage

The recommended dose of phenytoin is 100 milligrams every 5 minutes to a maximum loading dose of 1000 milligrams, until the arrhythmia is suppressed, or until symptoms of central nervous system depression appear.

Route

Phenytoin should be given by slow IV bolus with constant EKG monitoring.

How Supplied

Phenytoin (Dilantin®) is supplied in 2-milliliter ampules containing 100 milligrams of the drug. Dilantin is incompatible with solutions containing dextrose. If an infusion of Dilantin is prepared, the drug should be placed in normal saline.

Edrophonium chloride (Tensilon®)

Description

Tensilon belongs to a class of drugs referred to as **anticholinesterase agents**. Drugs in this group inhibit the actions of the enzyme **acetylcholinesterase**. This enzyme plays an important role in neurophysiology as it deactivates the neurotransmitter of the parasympathetic nervous system, acetylcholine. Physostigmine, an emergency drug used in the management of atropine-type poisonings and tricyclic antidepressant overdoses, is chemically similar to Tensilon. The neurophysiology of the parasympathetic nervous system is discussed in more detail in the following section on parasympatholytics.

Tensilon has proven effectiveness in the management of paroxysmal supraventricular tachycardias that do not respond to vagal maneuvers. The inhibition of acetylcholinesterase by Tensilon serves to enhance the acetylcholine secreted by the vagus nerve on the heart. This increased parasympathetic effect has been successful in terminating paroxysmal supraventricular tachycardias.

With the recent introduction of the slow calcium channel blockers (verapamil) and adenosine, Tensilon has fallen into disuse.

Indication

- PSVT refractory to vagal maneuvers

Contraindications

Tensilon should not be administered to patients with a history of hypersensitivity to the drug.

Precautions

The respiratory pattern should be carefully monitored during and following administration of Tensilon. Also, the patient should be constantly monitored for signs of bradycardia. Atropine sulfate should be readily available in those cases of bradycardia causing hemodynamic problems.

Do not administer Tensilon in dextrose solutions as it tends to crystalize in the tubing.

Dosage

The standard dosage is 5 milligrams initially intravenously. If unsuccessful after 10 minutes or so, a second dose of 10 milligrams may be administered.

Physicians frequently order the administration of a test dose of 0.1 to 0.5 milligrams before the administration of the full dose.

Route

Tensilon should be administered intravenously only.

How Supplied

Tensilon is supplied in ampules containing 10 milligrams of the drug in 1 milliliter of solvent.

Adenosine (Adenocard®)

Description

Adenosine (Adenocard®) is a naturally occurring substance that is present in all body cells. Adenosine decreases conduction of the electrical impulse through the AV node, which can effectively terminate rapid supraventricular arrhythmias such as PSVT. The half-life of adenosine is less than 10 seconds. Because of its rapid onset of action, and very short half-life, the administration of adenosine is sometimes referred to as "chemical cardioversion." A single bolus of the drug was effective in converting PSVT to a normal sinus rhythm in a significant number (>90%) of patients in the initial drug studies. Adenosine does not appear to cause hypotension to the same degree as does verapamil.

Indication

- PSVT (including that associated with Wolff-Parkinson-White syndrome) refractory to common vagal maneuvers

Contraindications

Adenosine is contraindicated in patients with second- or third-degree heart block, sick sinus syndrome, or those with known hypersensitivity to the drug.

Precautions

Adenosine will typically cause arrhythmias at the time of cardioversion. These will generally last a few seconds or less, and may include PVCs, premature atrial contractions, sinus bradycardia, sinus tachycardia, and

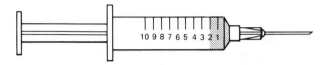

Figure 6–13   Administration of adenosine.

various degrees of AV block. In extreme cases, transient asystole may occur. If this occurs, appropriate therapy should be initiated.

Adenosine should be used cautiously in patients with asthma.

Common side effects occurring during adenosine administration include facial flushing, headache, shortness of breath, dizziness, and nausea, among others. Because the half-life of adenosine is so brief, side effects are generally self-limited.

Dosage

The initial dose of adenosine is 6 milligrams given as a rapid intravenous bolus over a 1- to 2-second period. To be certain that the drug rapidly reaches the central circulation it should be given directly into a vein or into a proximal medication port of a functioning IV line. It should be followed immediately by a rapid saline flush.

If the initial dose does not result in conversion of the PSVT within 1 to 2 minutes, a 12-milligram dose may be given as a rapid IV bolus. The 12-milligram dose may be repeated a second time if required. Doses greater than 12 milligrams should not be administered (see Figure 6–13).

Route

Adenosine should only be given by rapid IV bolus, directly into the vein, or into the medication administration port closest to the patient.

How Supplied

Adenosine (Adenocard®) is supplied in vials containing 6 milligrams of the drug in 2 milliliters of saline solvent.

PARASYMPATHOLYTICS

Drugs that inhibit the actions of the parasympathetic nervous system are referred to as **parasympatholytics**. Sometimes they are referred to as **anticholinergics**. To understand fully the role and actions of the sympathomimetics, we must first review the parasympathetic nervous system.

The parasympathetic, or **cholinergic** system, plays a major role in the maintenance of homeostasis. Parasympathetic stimulation induces peristalsis, causes pupillary constriction, and a decrease in the heart rate. The primary nerve of the parasympathetic nervous system is the **vagus nerve**.

The vagus nerve descends from the brain along the carotid arteries. It then innervates the heart and the digestive system. Paramedics should be familiar with the manual method of vagal stimulation, carotid sinus massage. Carotid sinus massage is used to slow the heart rate in paroxysmal supraventricular tachycardia.

When the vagus nerve is stimulated, it causes acetylcholine to be released from the presynaptic nerve endings. It then activates acetylcholine receptors on the target organs. These receptors cause the heart rate to slow. Then, after only a fraction of a second, cholinesterase is released, which deactivates acetylcholine. Several drugs act on this junction. The primary drug of this type is atropine sulfate. Atropine binds to the acetylcholine receptors, thus inhibiting activation. Besides increasing the heart rate, atropine is used frequently as a preoperative medication because it decreases digestive secretions, especially salivation. Certain chemicals, especially the organophosphate insecticides, tend to block, in an irreversible manner, the action of cholinesterase. Excessive levels of acetylcholine can cause serious problems.

Research has shown that some cases of asystole can be caused by an increase in parasympathetic tone. The reason for the increase is not clear. Based on this data, however, the American Heart Association recommends administering 1 milligram of atropine sulfate to any patient encountered in asystole as soon as possible.

Atropine Sulfate

Description

Atropine sulfate is a potent parasympatholytic. It blocks acetylcholine receptors, thus inhibiting parasympathetic stimulation. In emergency medicine, it is used primarily to increase the heart rate in life-threatening bradycardia. Although it has positive chronotropic properties, it has little or no inotropic effect. It plays an important role as an antidote in organophosphate poisonings.

Indications

- Bradycardias accompanied by hemodynamically significant hypotension or frequent ectopic escape beats; some use in treating second-degree Mobitz II and third-degree heart blocks in the setting of acute myocardial infarction
- Asystole

Contraindications

None in emergency situations.

Precautions

A maximum dose of 2 milligrams should not be exceeded, except in the setting of organophosphate poisoning. If the heart rate fails to increase after a total of 2 milligrams has been given, then isoproterenol or cardiac pacing is indicated.

Dosage

In the treatment of bradycardias, 0.5 milligram should be administered every 5 minutes until a maximum dose of 2.0 milligrams has been delivered.

In the treatment of asystole, the dose should be increased to 1.0 mg. When an IV cannot be placed, the dose can be administered endotracheally.

Route

Atropine should be given as an IV bolus in emergency situations.

How Supplied

Atropine is supplied in prefilled syringes containing 1.0 milligrams in 10 milliliters of solution.

CARDIAC GLYCOSIDES

Digitalis, the principal drug in the cardiac glycoside class, is one of the oldest medications known to humans. For hundreds of years it has been used in the treatment of congestive heart failure. Digitalis and the related cardiac glycosides increase the force (inotropic effect) of the myocardial contraction. When given to patients in congestive heart failure, it significantly increases the cardiac output, reducing left ventricular diameter, decreases venous pressure, and hastens reduction of peripheral and pulmonary edema. In recent years, digitalis has also proved effective in the management of patients with atrial flutter and atrial fibrillation. In these patients, rapid atrial rates produce accelerated ventricular rates, which can be reduced by digitalis therapy.

Several digitalis preparations are available. These include the following:

Digitoxin. Digitoxin is the longest-acting cardiac glycoside. It must not be confused with the shorter-acting digoxin.

Digoxin (Lanoxin®). Digoxin is the most commonly prescribed form of digitalis.

Ouabain. Ouabain has a rapid rate of onset and a relatively short duration of effect. Its use is reserved for cases in which rapid digitalization is required.

Deslanoside (Cedilanid-D®). Deslanoside is the most rapidly acting digitalis preparation.

Cardiac glycosides have profound effects on cardiac function and rhythm. The therapeutic index (therapeutic dose–toxic dose) is low, which means that the possibility of digitalis toxicity should always be considered in patients with this medication. Signs of digitalis toxicity include cardiac arrhythmias (PVCs, PSVT with 2:1 block, and so on), nausea, vomiting, headache, visual disturbances (yellow vision), and drowsiness. Almost any arrhythmia can be associated with digitalis toxicity.

Digitalis is a potent and potentially toxic drug. Extreme care must be used whenever it is administered. Constant monitoring of vital signs and EKG is essential. In almost all cases, digitalization should be deferred until the patient is in the emergency department and under the care of the emergency department physician.

Digoxin (Lanoxin®)

Description

Digoxin is a moderately rapid-acting cardiac glycoside. Therapeutic effects begin in about 0.5 hour and peak at 24 hours. It is effective in the treatment of congestive heart failure and rapid atrial arrhythmias. It significantly increases the stroke volume, thus increasing the cardiac output.

Indications

- Congestive heart failure
- Supraventricular tachyarrhythmias, especially atrial flutter and atrial fibrillation.

Contraindications

Digoxin should not be given to any patient showing any of the signs or symptoms of digitalis toxicity. It also should not be administered to patients in ventricular fibrillation.

Precautions

Patients receiving digoxin should be constantly monitored for signs and symptoms of digitalis toxicity. Extreme care should be used when administering digoxin to patients with myocardial infarction, as they are prone to digitalis toxicity. Digitalis toxicity is potentiated in patients with hypokalemia, hypomagnesemia, and hypercalcemia.

Dosage

The dosage is 0.25 to 0.5 milligrams given by slow IV push.

Route

Digoxin is generally given intravenously in the treatment of supraventricular tachyarrhythmias.

How Supplied

Digoxin (Lanoxin®) is supplied in 2-milliliter ampules containing 0.5 milligrams of the drug.

ALKALINIZING AGENTS

Alkalinizing drugs, such as sodium bicarbonate, are used to buffer the acids present in the body during and after severe hypoxia. Normal body pH is 7.4 (7.35 to 7.45). During hypoxia, serum pH may fall quickly. Sodium bicarbonate will help correct metabolic (usually lactic acid) acidosis until hypoxia is corrected. The following reaction illustrates the role of sodium bicarbonate in acid-base balance.

$$H^+ \; + \; HCO_3^- \; \rightleftharpoons H_2CO_3 \rightleftharpoons H_2O \; + \; CO_2$$

Acids	Bicarbonate	Carbonic	Water	Carbon
(Strong)		Acid		Dioxide
		(Weak)		

Bicarbonate combines with the strong acids, usually lactic acid, and forms a weak, volatile acid. This acid then is broken down into carbon dioxide and water. The two end products are then removed via the lungs and the kidneys.

Excessive administration of sodium bicarbonate may cause metabolic alkalosis, which may be worse than the metabolic acidosis being treated.

Primary treatment of metabolic acidosis in the setting of hypoxia or cardiac arrest is adequate oxygenation and blood pressure support.

Sodium Bicarbonate

Description

For many years sodium bicarbonate was the cornerstone of advanced cardiac life support care. Controlled studies showed that sodium bicarbonate was ineffective in the treatment of cardiac arrest, however, and was actually associated with many adverse reactions.

Sodium bicarbonate is occasionally used in the treatment of certain types of drug overdose. The most common example is drugs in the tricyclic class of antidepressants. Overdosage of these drugs has serious effects including life-threatening cardiac arrhythmias. Tricyclic antidepressant excretion from the body is enhanced by making the urine more alkaline (raising the pH). Sodium bicarbonate is sometimes administered to increase the pH of the urine to speed excretion of the drug from the body.

Indications

- Late in the management of cardiac arrest, if at all. Hyperventilation, prompt defibrillation, and the administration of epinephrine and lidocaine should always precede use of sodium bicarbonate. Because these therapies take at least 10 minutes to carry out, sodium bicarbonate should never be administered in the first 10 minutes of a resuscitation.
- Tricyclic antidepressant overdose
- Severe acidosis refractory to hyperventilation

Contraindications

When used in the management of the situations described earlier, there are no absolute contraindications.

Precautions

Sodium bicarbonate can cause metabolic alkalosis when administered in large quantities. It is important to calculate the dosage based on patient weight and size.

Most vasopressors can be deactivated by alkaline solutions like sodium bicarbonate.

Sodium bicarbonate should not be administered in conjunction with calcium chloride. A precipitate will form, which may clog the IV line.

Dosage

The correct dose of sodium bicarbonate is 1 milliequivalent per kilogram of body weight initially followed by 0.5 milliequivalent per kilogram body weight every 10 minutes. When possible, the dosage of sodium bicarbonate should be based on the results of arterial blood gas studies.

Route

Sodium bicarbonate should be administered only as an IV bolus.

How Supplied

Sodium bicarbonate comes in prefilled syringes containing 50 milli-equivalents of the drug in 50 milliliters of solvent.

ANALGESICS

Drugs that have proved to be effective in alleviating pain are referred to as **analgesics**. Although they may be administered in many different types of emergencies, they are usually reserved for the treatment of emergencies involving the cardiovascular system, especially myocardial infarction.

As a rule, undiagnosed pain is usually not treated. Early administration of analgesics to these patients may alter physical findings and impair emergency evaluation by the emergency physician. Some types of pain may be easy to distinguish and are sometimes treated in the prehospital setting. These include chest pain associated with acute myocardial infarction, severe burns, and kidney stones.

Analgesics include the following:

- Morphine sulfate
- Meperidine (Demerol®)
- Nalbuphine (Nubain®)
- Nitronox®
- Nitrous oxide
- Butorphanol tartrate (Stadol®)

Morphine is derived from the opium plant. It has impressive analgesic and hemodynamic effects. Meperidine, although similar to morphine in its analgesic effects, is considerably different chemically and is synthetically derived. Nalbuphine (Nubain®) is also a potent synthetic analgesic. It does not have the hemodynamic effects that morphine does, yet it is often used in emergency medicine because it does not cause respiratory depression and has a low tendency for abuse. Stadol®, another of the new breed of synthetic analgesics, is similar to Nubain but is rarely used in treating cardiovascular emergencies. Nitronox®, a 50% mixture of oxygen and nitrous oxide that can be easily inhaled by the patient, is entirely different from the other analgesic agents discussed. Its analgesic effects are also very potent, yet disappear within a few minutes after the cessation of administration. Thus, Nitronox can be given for many types of pain in the field without fear of impairing subsequent physical examination in the emergency department. In addition to its analgesic effects, Nitronox delivers oxygen to the patient, which makes it useful in cardiac emergencies.

Morphine Sulfate

Description

Although morphine sulfate is one of the most potent analgesics known to humans, it also has hemodynamic properties that make it extremely useful in emergency medicine. It increases peripheral venous capacitance and decreases venous return. This effect is sometimes called a "chemical phlebotomy." Morphine also decreases myocardial oxygen demand. This action is due to both the decreased systemic vascular resistance and the sedative effects of the drug. Patient apprehension and fear can significantly increase myocardial oxygen demand, and in some cases can conceivably increase the size of myocardial infarction. The hemodynamic properties of morphine make it one of the most important drugs used in the treatment of pulmonary edema. Morphine is frequently administered to patients with signs and symptoms of pulmonary edema who are not having chest pain.

Morphine is a narcotic derivative of opium. It has a high tendency for addiction and abuse and is thus covered under the **Controlled Substances Act** of 1970. It is classified as a Schedule II drug. Because of this, there are special considerations involved in the handling of the drug. Many emergency medical services (EMS) systems have opted to use the synthetic analgesics, like nalbuphine and pentazocine, instead of morphine and meperidine because of these problems.

Morphine causes severe respiratory depression in higher doses. This is especially true in patients who already have some form of respiratory impairment. The narcotic antagonist naloxone (Narcan®) should be readily available whenever the drug is administered.

Indications

- Severe pain associated with myocardial infarction, kidney stones, and so on
- Pulmonary edema either with or without associated pain

Contraindications

Morphine should not be used in patients who are volume depleted or severely hypotensive because of the hemodynamic effects described earlier. Morphine should not be administered to any patient with a history of hypersensitivity to the drug, or to patients with undiagnosed head injury or abdominal pain.

Precautions

Morphine can cause respiratory depression. The paramedic should always have naloxone available to reverse the effects of the drug if respiratory depression ensues. Patients who are extremely ill, or who may have preexisting respiratory depression, may be extremely sensitive to the depressive effects of morphine.

Dosage

There are many different approaches to the administration of morphine. An initial dose in the range of 2 to 10 milligrams intravenously is standard. This can be augmented with additional doses of 2 milligrams every few minutes and can be continued until the pain is relieved or until signs of respiratory depression occur.

Intramuscular injection usually requires 5 to 15 milligrams based on the patient's weight to attain desired effects.

Routes

Morphine is routinely given intravenously in emergency medicine. It can also be given intramuscularly, however.

How Supplied

Morphine comes in tamper-proof ampules and Tubex® prefilled cartridges. To ease administration, the 10 milligrams in 1-milliliter dilution is preferred.

Meperidine (Demerol®)

Description

Meperidine is extensively used in medicine for the treatment of moderate to severe pain. It is less potent than morphine sulfate. Sixty to 80 milligrams of meperidine are equivalent in action to 10 milligrams of morphine. It does not have the same hemodynamic properties but has the same tendency for physical dependence and abuse. Because it causes respiratory depression, naloxone should be available whenever meperidine is administered. The rate of onset is slightly faster than morphine, yet its effects are much shorter in duration. Like morphine, meperidine is a Schedule II drug regulated under the **Controlled Substances Act** of 1970.

Indication

- Moderate to severe pain

Contraindications

Meperidine should not be administered to patients who are receiving, or who have recently received monoamine oxidase inhibitors (for example, Nardil®, Parnate®, and Eutron®). Therapeutic doses of meperidine have occasionally caused severe, and sometimes fatal, reactions in patients receiving these agents.

It also should not be administered to patients with undiagnosed abdominal pain or head injury.

Precautions

Meperidine can cause respiratory depression. The paramedic should always have naloxone available to reverse the effects of the drug if respiratory depression ensues. Like morphine, meperidine should be kept in a secure locked box.

Dosage

The usual dose used in the treatment of severe pain is 50 to 100 milligrams intramuscularly or intravenously.

Routes

Meperidene can be administered either intravenously or intramuscularly.

How Supplied

Meperidene (Demerol®) is supplied in ampules and Tubex® prefilled cartridges containing 50 milligrams of the drug in 1 milliliter of solvent.

Nitrous Oxide (Nitronox®)

Description

Nitronox is a blended mixture of 50 percent nitrous and 50 percent oxygen. When inhaled, it has potent analgesic effects. These quickly dissipate, however, within 2 to 5 minutes after cessation of administration.

The Nitronox unit consists of one oxygen and one nitrous oxide cylinder. The gases are fed into a blender that combines them at the appropriate concentration. The mixture is then delivered to a modified demand valve for administration to the patient.

Nitronox must be self-administered. It is effective in treating many varieties of pain encountered in the prehospital setting including pain from many types of trauma. The high concentration of oxygen delivered along with the nitrous oxide will increase the oxygen tension in the blood, thus reducing hypoxia.

Indications

- Pain of musculoskeletal origin, particularly fractures
- Burns
- Suspected ischemic chest pain
- States of severe anxiety including hyperventilation

Contraindications

Nitronox should not be used in any patient who cannot comprehend verbal instructions or those intoxicated with alcohol or other drugs. It should not be administered to any patient with a head injury who exhibits an altered mental status. Nitronox should not be administered to any patient with COPD where the high concentration of oxygen (50 percent) might result in respiratory depression. Nitrous oxide tends to diffuse into closed spaces more readily than either carbon dioxide or oxygen. Many COPD patients have air-containing blebs in their lungs, and nitrous oxide can concentrate in these blebs causing them to swell. Swollen blebs may rupture causing a pneumothorax.

Nitronox should not be administered to patients with a thoracic injury suspicious of pneumothorax as the gas may accumulate in the pneumothorax increasing its size. Also, patients with severe abdominal pain and distention, suggestive of bowel obstruction, should not receive Nitronox. Nitrous oxide can concentrate in pockets of obstructed bowel possibly leading to rupture.

Precautions

Nitronox should only be used in areas that are well ventilated. When the gas is used in the patient compartment of an ambulance it is recommended that a scavenging system be in place.

Nitrous oxide exists in a liquid state inside the gas cylinder. Heat present in the air, the cylinder wall, or the various regulators and lines causes the liquid to vaporize. This vaporization process makes the cylinder tank and lines cool to touch. Following prolonged use, frost may develop on the cylinder, regulator, or lines. In very cold environments, generally less than 21°F (−6°C), the liquid may be slow to vaporize, and administration may be impossible.

Dosage

Nitronox should only be self-administered. Continuous administration may take place until the pain is significantly relieved, or the patient drops the mask. The patient care record should document the duration of drug administration.

Nalbuphine (Nubain®)

Description

Nalbuphine is a recent addition to the analgesic group. It is a synthetic drug with a potency equivalent to morphine on a milligram to milligram basis. Its onset of action is considerably faster than morphine, occurring within 2 to 3 minutes after intravenous administration. Its duration of effect is reported to be 3 to 6 hours. Although nalbuphine causes some respiratory depression in doses up to 10 milligrams, these effects do not seem to get worse in doses that exceed 10 milligrams. Naloxone is an effective antagonist and should be available when nalbuphine is administered.

At this time, nalbuphine is not regulated under the **Controlled Substances Act**. Current studies show that it has a minimal tendency for physical dependence and abuse. This property has made nalbuphine increasingly popular in prehospital care.

Indication

- Moderate to severe pain

Contraindications

Nalbuphine should not be administered to patients with head injury or undiagnosed abdominal pain.

Precautions

The primary precaution in using nalbuphine is in patients with impaired respiratory function. Small doses of nalbuphine may cause significant respiratory depression. Naloxone should be readily available. Nalbuphine also has narcotic antagonistic properties. Thus, it should be administered with caution to patients dependent on narcotics as it may cause withdrawal effects.

Dosage

The general regimen for nalbuphine administration is 5 milligrams intravenously initially. This may be augmented with additional 2 milligrams doses if necessary.

Route

Nalbuphine can be administered intravenously or intramuscularly.

How Supplied

Nalbuphine is supplied in 1-milliliter ampules containing 10 milligrams of the drug.

Butorphanol Tartrate (Stadol®)

Description

Butorphanol, one of the new breed of synthetic analgesics, is starting to receive extensive use in emergency medicine. It is quite potent; the analgesic effects of 2 milligrams of butorphanol are equivalent to 10 milligrams of morphine. Although butorphanol can cause respiratory depression, this effect usually plateaus following administration of approximately 4 milligrams. Currently, butorphanol is not restricted under the **Controlled Substances Act**. This makes it quite attractive for use in the prehospital phase of emergency medical care.

Like nalbuphine, butorphanol has some narcotic antagonistic properties. Caution should be used when administering butorphanol to patients already dependent on narcotics.

Although we have chosen to discuss butorphanol along with the other prehospital analgesics in the cardiovascular emergencies chapter, it is rarely used in treating chest pain accompanying myocardial infarction. Its use is primarily reserved for general musculoskeletal and soft-tissue pain, such as that which accompanies fractures and burns.

Indication

- Moderate to severe pain

Contraindications

Butorphanol should not be administered to any patient with a history of hypersensitivity to the drug. Also, it should not be given to patients dependent on narcotics as it may well cause some reversal of the narcotic effects. It should not be administered to patients with head injury or undiagnosed abdominal pain.

Precautions

If butorphanol causes marked respiratory depression, then Narcan® can be administered to reverse its effects. Remember, when administering any potent analgesic, it is possible to mask other signs and symptoms, thus delaying the complete physical examination and determination of a diagnosis. All analgesics should be administered only after a thorough physical examination.

Butorphanol should not be administered to any patient with head injury as it may well cause an increase in cerebrospinal pressure.

Dosage

The standard dose of butorphanol is 1 milligram intravenously every 3 to 4 hours. When given intramuscularly the standard dose is 2 milligrams.

Route

Butorphanol should only be administered intravenously or intramuscularly.

How Supplied

Butorphanol is supplied in 2-milliliter vials containing 2 milligrams of the drug.

DIURETICS

One of the more common cardiovascular emergencies that emergency personnel are called on to treat is congestive heart failure. Congestive heart failure occurs when the heart loses its ability to pump blood effectively. When this occurs, the venous vessels leading to the heart become engorged. Failure of the left side of the heart causes a buildup of blood in the pulmonary circulation. Failure of the right side of the heart results in congestion of the peripheral circulation, which usually manifests as peripheral edema. Common signs of right heart failure include jugular venous distention, ascites, and pedal (ankle or pretibial) edema.

In the treatment of congestive heart failure, the primary objectives are to increase the cardiac output and to reduce pulmonary and peripheral edema. Although the inotropic effects of digitalis preparation will increase cardiac output, the rate of onset is relatively slow, making this drug less than ideal in acute pulmonary edema. In acute heart failure, the most effective therapy is to reduce venous filling pressure. This can be done mechanically by applying rotating tourniquets, which are placed on three of the extremities to decrease venous return. Phlebotomy (drawing blood out of the circulatory system) can also be employed. The *preferred* method, however, is the administration of potent diuretics.

Furosemide (Lasix®)

Description

Furosemide is a potent diuretic that inhibits sodium chloride reabsorption in the kidney and that causes venous dilatation. It is extremely useful in the treatment of congestive heart failure and pulmonary edema. Its effects are usually evident within 5 minutes of administration.

Indications

- Congestive heart failure
- Pulmonary edema

Contraindications

Usage in pregnancy should be limited to life-threatening situations in which the benefits of furosemide outweigh the risks. Furosemide has been known to cause fetal abnormalities.

Precautions

Dehydration and electrolyte depletion can result from excessive doses of potent diuretics. Furosemide should be protected from light.

Dosage

The standard dosage of furosemide is 40 milligrams given by slow IV push in patients already on chronic oral furosemide therapy, and 20 milligrams intravenously in patients who are not taking the drug orally on a regular basis. Dosages as high as 80 milligrams intravenously may be indicated in severe cases.

Route

Furosemide should be given intravenously in emergency situations.

How Supplied

Furosemide is supplied in ampules and prefilled syringes. These containers contain 10 milligrams per milliliter.

Bumetanide (Bumex®)

Description

Bumetanide is a potent diuretic with a rapid rate of onset and a short duration of action. Like furosemide, bumetanide inhibits the reabsorption of sodium chloride in the kidneys.

Indications

- Congestive heart failure
- Pulmonary edema

Contraindications

Usage in pregnancy should be limited to life-threatening situations in which the benefits of using bumetanide outweigh the risks.

Precautions

Dehydration and electrolyte depletion can result from excessive doses of potent diuretics. Patients who have experienced allergic reactions to furosemide have not experienced those same reactions when administered bumetanide, which suggests that this drug may be used in patients with furosemide allergy who are in need of rapid diuresis.

Dosage

The usual initial dose of bumetanide is 0.5 to 1.0 milligram given during a period of 1 to 2 minutes. A second or third dose can be administered at 2- to 3-hour intervals if required. The total daily dosage should not exceed 10 milligrams.

Route

Bumetanide injection can be given by either the IV or intramuscular routes. In the emergency setting, the IV route is preferred.

How Supplied

Bumetanide (Bumex®) is supplied in ampules containing 0.5 milligrams in 2 milliliters of solvent (0.25 milligrams per milliliter). It is also supplied in 2-, 4-, and 10-milliliter vials containing 0.25 milligrams per milliliter.

ANTIANGINAL AGENTS

A common manifestation of advanced cardiovascular disease is angina pectoris, which results from narrowing of the coronary arteries resulting from the buildup of atherosclerotic plaques, or coronary artery vasospasm. In exercise, and other stressful situations, the amount of blood that can be carried by the coronary arteries may not be sufficient to meet the oxygen demands of the myocardium. This results in myocardial hypoxia, causing the classic pain syndrome called angina pectoris. Sublingual nitroglycerin usually gives immediate relief by causing dilatation of the coronary arteries and decreased cardiac work. In recent years there have been trials in which nitroglycerin has been administered to patients suffering myocardial infarction in the hope of decreasing the extent of myocardial damage. Nitroglycerin is often administered to patients complaining of chest pain to rule out angina as the cause. When cardiac pain is not relieved by nitroglycerin, morphine and other potent analgesics are administered.

Nitroglycerin is usually administered sublingually. Recently, however, it has been given intravenously in some cases of unstable angina and acute myocardial infarction.

Calcium ion antagonists, such as nifedipine (Procardia®), have proved effective in the management of angina, especially that believed owing to coronary artery vasospasm.

Nitroglycerin (Nitro Stat®)

Description

Nitroglycerin is a rapid smooth-muscle relaxant that causes decreased cardiac work, and to a lesser degree, vasodilatation of coronary arteries, thus increasing perfusion of the ischemic myocardium. Pain relief occurs within 1 to 2 minutes, and therapeutic effects can be observed up to 30 minutes later.

Indications

- Chest pain associated with angina pectoris
- Chest pain associated with acute myocardial infarction
- Acute pulmonary edema (unless accompanied by hypotension)

Contraindications

Nitroglycerin is contraindicated in patients who are hypotensive or who may have increased intracranial pressure.

Precautions

Patients taking nitroglycerin may develop a tolerance for the drug, which necessitates increasing the dose. Headache is a common side effect of nitroglycerin administration and results from vasodilation of cerebral vessels. Nitroglycerin deteriorates quite rapidly once the bottle is opened. When a bottle of nitroglycerin is opened, it should be dated. Nitroglycerin should also be protected from light.

Always monitor the blood pressure during nitroglycerin administration.

Dosage

One tablet (0.4 milligram) sublingually for routine angina pectoris. This can be repeated as required.

Routes

Nitroglycerin should be administered sublingually. Care should be taken to assure that it is not swallowed. IV nitroglycerin is receiving some use in emergency departments and intensive care units, but the sublingual route is adequate for most prehospital situations. Nitroglycerin is also available in patches and in ointment form for transdermal administration.

How Supplied

Nitroglycerin is supplied in bottles containing 0.4 milligram tablets (1/150 grain). The tablets must be protected from light and air to prevent deterioration.

Nitropaste (Nitro-Bid® Ointment)

Description

Nitropaste contains a 2% solution of nitroglycerin in a special absorbent paste. When placed on the skin, nitroglycerin is absorbed into the systemic circulation. In many cases, nitropaste may be preferred over nitroglycerin tablets because of its longer duration of action.

Indications

- Chest pain associated with angina pectoris
- Chest pain associated with acute myocardial infarction

Contraindications

Nitropaste is contraindicated in patients with increased intracranial pressure. It should not be administered to patients who are hypotensive.

Precautions

Patients taking the drug routinely may develop a tolerance for the drug and require an increased dose. Headache is a common side effect of nitroglycerin administration and occurs as a result of vasodilatation of the cerebral vessels.

Postural syncope sometimes occurs following the administration of nitroglycerin. This should be anticipated and the patient kept supine when possible. It is important to monitor the blood pressure constantly.

Dosage

Generally ½ to ¾ inch (1 to 2 centimeter) of the nitropaste is applied. Measuring applicators are supplied.

How Supplied

Nitropaste is supplied in 20-gram and 60-gram tubes. Several dose-measuring applicators are also included.

Nitroglycerin Spray (Nitrolingual® Spray)

Description

Nitroglycerin spray is a special preparation of nitroglycerin in an aerosol form that delivers precisely 0.4 milligram of nitroglycerin per spray. Peak effects following administration occur within 4 minutes.

Indications

- Chest pain associated with angina pectoris
- Chest pain associated with acute myocardial infarction

Contraindications

Nitroglycerin is contraindicated in patients who are hypotensive or who may have increased intracranial pressure.

Precautions

Patients taking nitroglycerin routinely may develop a tolerance for the drug. Headache is a common side effect of nitroglycerin administration and results from dilation of cerebral blood vessels. This should be anticipated. The blood pressure should be monitored during nitroglycerin therapy.

Dosage

One spray (0.4 milligram) should be sprayed under the tongue at the onset of an attack of angina. No more than three sprays are recommended in a 25-minute period. *The spray should not be inhaled.*

Route

Nitroglycerin spray should be applied to the sublingual mucous membranes in the manner described earlier.

How Supplied

Nitroglycerin spray is supplied in an aerosol container containing 200 doses of nitroglycerin.

ANTIHYPERTENSIVES

A dangerously elevated blood pressure is a hypertensive emergency. A **hypertensive crisis** is defined as a sudden increase in the systolic and diastolic blood pressure causing a functional disturbance of the central nervous system, the heart, or the kidneys. Hypertensive emergencies call for prompt and efficient care by prehospital providers.

Hypertensive emergencies are often divided into two categories: hypertensive emergencies and hypertensive urgencies. A **hypertensive emergency** is a situation in which the blood pressure must be lowered within 1 hour. A **hypertensive urgency** is a situation in which the blood pressure should be lowered within 24 hours. Hypertensive emergencies develop when the blood pressure exceeds 130 millimeters of mercury diastolic. It can be complicated by hypertensive encephalopathy, acute pulmonary edema, stroke, or acute myocardial ischemia. Nose bleed, or epistaxis, is also common. **Hypertensive encephalopathy** is the most devastating complication of hypertension. Signs and symptoms include severe headache, nausea and vomiting, and an altered mental state. This can range from lethargy or confusion to coma. Neurological symptoms may be present as well. These can include blindness, inability to speak, muscle twitches, weakness, or paralysis. The treatment is to lower blood pressure as rapidly and as safely as possible.

There are several agents available to lower blood pressure acutely. The most popular of these is nifedipine (Procardia®). Procardia can be administered sublingually with an onset of action in less than 10 minutes. In hypertension refractory to nifedipine, sodium nitroprusside is often used. Sodium nitroprusside is administered as a controlled infusion that can be titrated to obtain the desired pressure. Hydralazine is often used to lower the blood pressure in pregnancy to prevent eclampsia. Diazoxide

(Hyperstat®), once used commonly in emergency care, has fallen into relative disuse with nifedipine being the preferred agent.

Nifedipine (Procardia®)

Description

Nifedipine is a calcium channel blocker that is receiving widespread usage in emergency medicine. Nifedipine causes relaxation of the smooth muscles that encircle the peripheral blood vessels, principally the arterioles. This relaxation results in peripheral vasodilation, decreased peripheral vascular resistance, and a decrease in both the systolic and diastolic blood pressure. Nifedipine is also effective in reducing coronary artery spasm in angina.

Indications

- Severe hypertension
- Angina pectoris

Contraindications

Nifedipine is contraindicated in patients with known hypersensitivity to the drug. It should not be administered to patients who are hypotensive.

Precautions

Nifedipine can cause a significant drop in blood pressure. Thus, the blood pressure should be frequently monitored. Nifedipine should be used with caution in patients with heart failure. *Nifedipine should not be administered to patients receiving IV β blockers.*

Dosage

One 10-milligram capsule should have several small puncture holes placed in the capsule and then placed under the tongue where it can be absorbed. Alternatively, the capsule can be bitten by the patient and swallowed with approximately the same rate of onset.

Route

Nifedipine should only be administered orally or sublingually as described earlier.

How Supplied

Nifedipine is supplied in 10- and 20-milligram tablets.

Sodium Nitroprusside (Nitropress®, Nipride®)

Description

Sodium nitroprusside is a potent vasodilating agent used in the management of hypertensive crisis when a prompt reduction in blood pressure is required. It acts by dilating both peripheral arteries and peripheral veins. This results in an immediate reduction in blood pressure, which is generally proportional to the rate of drug administration. Sodium nitroprusside administration is usually accompanied by an increase in heart rate.

Although not approved, sodium nitroprusside is occasionally used in the management of severe congestive heart failure. The dilation of the peripheral veins results in decreased blood return to the heart (preload). In addition, the dilation of the peripheral arteries reduces the pressure against which the heart has to pump (afterload). This results in a net increase in cardiac output in patients with severe congestive heart failure (see Figure 6–14).

Because sodium nitroprusside is such a potent agent, the blood pressure, pulse rate, respiratory status, and EKG should be constantly monitored during drug administration.

Indication

- Hypertensive crisis in which a prompt reduction in blood pressure is essential

Contraindications

None when used in the management of life-threatening hypertensive crisis.

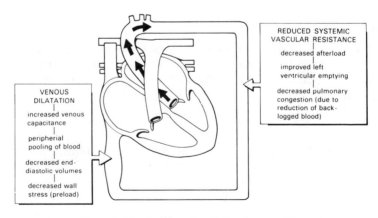

Figure 6–14   Actions of sodium nitroprusside.

Precautions

Once the sodium nitroprusside infusion is prepared it should be immediately wrapped in an opaque material, usually aluminum foil, to protect it from light. Once exposed to light the drug is quickly inactivated.

Sodium nitroprusside should not be used in children or pregnant women in the prehospital setting. The dosage should be reduced somewhat in elderly patients. The constant monitoring of blood pressure and pulse is essential throughout sodium nitroprusside administration.

Dosage

Fifty milligrams of sodium nitroprusside should be diluted in 500 milliliters of D_5W. This will give a concentration of 100 micrograms per milliliter. The initial dose should be 0.5 micrograms per kilogram per minute (see Figure 6–15).

Route

Sodium nitroprusside should only be diluted in D_5W and administered by slow IV infusion using a minidrip administration set. *This medication should never be given by IV bolus.*

How Supplied

Sodium nitroprusside is supplied in 5-milliliter vials containing 50 milligrams of the drug. Sodium nitroprusside is supplied in 2-milliliter vials containing 50 milligrams of the drug.

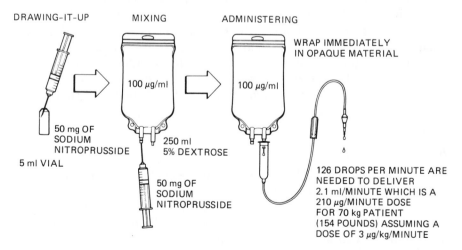

Figure 6–15   Preparation of sodium nitroprusside infusion.

Hydralazine (Apresoline®)

Description

Hydralazine, like sodium nitroprusside, is a potent vasodilating agent used to lower blood pressure in cases of hypertensive crisis. Hydralazine relaxes vascular smooth muscle, primarily in the arterial system, thus causing decreased arterial pressure (diastolic greater than systolic), decreased peripheral resistance, and increased cardiac output. Hydralazine causes postural hypotension to a lesser degree than sodium nitroprusside. The effects of hydralazine are usually seen within 5 to 10 minutes after the initiation of therapy.

Indications

- Hypertensive crisis in which a prompt reduction in blood pressure is required
- Hypertension complicating pregnancy (preeclampsia)

Contraindications

Hydralazine should not be administered to patients with a known history of coronary artery disease, rheumatic heart disease involving the mitral valve, or in any patient with a history of hypersensitivity to the drug.

Precautions

The administration of hydralazine may cause angina pectoris or EKG changes because of the increased cardiac output. This drug should not be used in the prehospital phase of emergency medical care to children because of limited experience with the drug in these cases. The blood pressure, pulse rate, respiratory status, and EKG should be monitored at all times during hydralazine therapy. Headache, nausea, and vomiting have been known to occur following hydralazine therapy and should be expected.

Dosage

The usual dosage of hydralazine in the management of hypertensive crisis is 20 to 40 milligrams given by slow IV bolus. This can be repeated, if required. If an IV line cannot be established, then the same dosage of the drug can be given by intramuscular injection. The blood pressure and EKG should be continuously monitored.

Route

Parenteral hydralazine should be administered by slow IV bolus. When necessary, however, the drug can be administered by intramuscular injection.

How Supplied

Hydralazine is supplied in 1-milliliter ampules containing 20 milligrams of the drug.

Diazoxide (Hyperstat®)

Description

Diazoxide is effective in the treatment of hypertensive crisis. It causes a decrease in both systolic and diastolic pressure by causing vasodilatation of the peripheral arterioles.

Indication

- Malignant hypertension in which a prompt decrease in diastolic blood pressure is indicated

Contraindications

Although there are some medical conditions for which diazoxide is contraindicated, the paramedic will most likely be unaware of these in the field.

Precautions

Hypotension may occur, and if severe, should be treated with sympathomimetics. Because of the rapid onset of action of diazoxide, frequent blood pressure monitoring (every minute) to detect possible hypotension is mandatory.

Dosage

The standard dose of diazoxide is 1 to 3 milligrams per kilogram given intravenously over 30 seconds up to 150 milligrams per kilogram. The dose may be repeated at 5- to 15-minute intervals as required.

Route

Diazoxide is administered intravenously.

How Supplied

Diazoxide is supplied in ampules containing 300 milligrams of the drug in 20 milliliters of solvent.

OTHER CARDIOVASCULAR DRUGS

The following agent does not readily fit into the classes of drugs discussed thus far.

Calcium Chloride

Description

Calcium chloride causes a significant increase in the myocardial contractile force and appears to increase ventricular automaticity. Although frequently used for many years in the management of cardiac arrest, especially that resulting from asystole and electromechanical dissociation, recent studies have presented data that seriously question the role of calcium chloride, even in these situations.

Indications

- Acute hyperkalemia (elevated potassium)
- Acute hypocalcemia (decreased calcium)
- Calcium-channel–blocker toxicity (nifedipine, verapamil, and so on)

Contraindications

Caution is warranted when calcium chloride is administered to patients receiving digitalis, as it may precipitate digitalis toxicity.

Precautions

It is extremely important to flush the IV line between administrations of calcium chloride and sodium bicarbonate to avoid precipitation.

Dosage

The standard dose for calcium chloride is 2 to 4 milligrams per kilogram intravenously. This may be repeated every 10 minutes as required.

Route

Calcium chloride should only be given intravenously.

How Supplied

Calcium chloride comes in prefilled syringes containing 1 gram of the drug in 10 milliliters of solvent (10 milliliters of a 10% solution).

SUMMARY

All of the medications discussed in this chapter are only of value when used in conjunction with other treatment modalities. Without appropriate cardiopulmonary resuscitation, the medications used in the management of cardiac arrest are not effective.

As mentioned, the dosages presented in this chapter are based on nationally accepted regimens. You should become familiar with the routine dosages and protocols used in your area.

7

DRUGS USED IN TREATMENT OF RESPIRATORY EMERGENCIES

INTRODUCTION

Oxygen is the most commonly used drug in the management of respiratory emergencies. In addition to oxygen, however, several pharmacologic agents have proved quite effective in relieving respiratory distress. In this chapter, medications used in the prehospital phase of emergency medical care are discussed.

Sympathomimetics are the most common agents used in the treatment of respiratory emergencies. The principal sympathomimetics include epinephrine, isoetharine, and terbutaline. In treating cardiovascular emergencies it is highly desirable to activate β_1 adrenergic receptors. When treating patients in respiratory distress, however, it is desirable to activate β_2 receptors. Unfortunately, most of the agents that activate β_2 receptors also have some effect on β_1 receptors. When activated, β_1 receptors cause an increase in heart rate and myocardial contractile force; β_2 receptors cause peripheral vasodilation, and most important, bronchodilation. Common side effects include palpitations, anxiety, and dizziness. Considerable effort has been devoted to isolation of pharmacological agents that act principally on β_2 receptors. Currently, sympathomimetic agents used in the prehospital phase of emergency medical care are chemically related to epinephrine but tend to be more selective for β_2 receptors than epinephrine.

Another agent used in the management of respiratory emergencies is **aminophylline**. Aminophylline, chemically unrelated to the catecholamines, belongs to a class of drugs called **xanthines**. A commonly encountered drug within the xanthines class is caffeine. Aminophylline causes relaxation of the bronchiole smooth musculature.

Epinephrine 1 : 1000

Description

Epinephrine 1:1000 is given subcutaneously to ensure a steady and prolonged action. It is sometimes used for treating the bronchoconstriction accompanying asthma and is also effective in treating bronchoconstriction associated with anaphylaxis.

Indications (Respiratory)

- Bronchial asthma
- Exacerbation of some forms of COPD
- Anaphylaxis

Contraindications

Because of the cardiac effects seen with the administration of epinephrine, it should not be administered to patients with underlying cardiovascular disease or hypertension.

Precautions

Epinephrine should be protected from light. Also, as with the other catecholamines, it tends to be deactivated by alkaline solutions. Any patient receiving epinephrine 1:1000 should be carefully monitored for changes in blood pressure, pulse, and EKG. Palpitations, anxiety, nausea, and headache are fairly common side effects.

Dosage

The standard dose of epinephrine 1:1000 ranges from 0.3 to 0.5 milligram depending on patient weight and condition, with 0.3 milligram being the usual starting dose. In the prehospital phase of emergency medical care, epinephrine 1:1000 should only be administered subcutaneously.

Route

Epinephrine 1:1000 should only be administered subcutaneously.

How Supplied

Epinephrine is supplied in ampules and prefilled syringes containing 1 milligram of the drug in 1 milliliter of solvent.

Epinephrine Suspension (Sus-Phrine®)

Description

Sus-Phrine® has the same pharmacological properties as epinephrine. Approximately 80 percent of the epinephrine present in Sus-Phrine, however, is in suspension. The epinephrine in solution, approximately 0.5 milligram, causes immediate bronchodilation, whereas prolonged action is obtained from the remaining epinephrine that is in the suspension. It is released slowly, maintaining therapeutic levels for 3 to 6 hours. Sus-Phrine® is usually administered just before discharge from the emergency department after the patient has been initially treated with epinephrine 1:1000.

Indication

- Bronchial asthma

Contraindications

Sus-Phrine® should not be administered to patients with underlying cardiovascular disease or hypertension.

Precautions

Sus-Phrine®, like any other epinephrine preparation, may cause tachycardia, anxiety, and dizziness. The patient's vital signs must be constantly monitored.

Dosage

The standard adult dosage is 0.1 to 0.3 milliliter of the 1:200 dilution, or one-half the epinephrine 1:1000 dose used in the initial treatment.

Route

Sus-Phrine® should be only administered subcutaneously.

How Supplied

Sus-Phrine® is supplied in 0.5-milliliter ampules of a 1:200 solution.

Racemic Epinephrine (microNEFRIN®, Vaponefrin®)

Description

Racemic epinephrine is slightly different chemically from the epinephrine compounds that have been discussed previously. Compounds that differ only in their chemical arrangement are called **isomers**. This particular form is frequently used in children to treat croup.

Racemic epinephrine should only be administered by inhalation.

Indication

* Croup (laryngotracheobronchitis)

Contraindications

Racemic epinephrine should not be used in the management of epiglottitis.

Precautions

Racemic epinephrine can result in tachycardia and possibly arrhythmias. Vital signs should be monitored.

Dosage

A concentration of 1:1000 (7.5 to 15 milliliters) is the standard dosage. It should only be used initially and not repeated.

Route

Racemic epinephrine should be given only by inhalation, generally by small-volume nebulizer, diluted with 2 to 3 milliliters of normal saline.

How Supplied

Racemic epinephrine is supplied in inhalator or nebulizer bottles containing either 7.5, 15, or 30 milliliters.

Terbutaline (Brethine®)

Description

Terbutaline is a synthetic sympathomimetic that is selective for β_2-adrenergic receptors. It causes immediate bronchodilation with minimal cardiac effects. Its onset of action is similar to that of epinephrine.

Indications

- Bronchial asthma
- Reversible bronchospasm associated with chronic bronchitis and emphysema

Contraindications

Terbutaline should not be administered to any patient with a history of hypersensitivity to the drug.

Precautions

Palpitations, anxiety, nausea, and dizziness may be seen following the administration of terbutaline. As with any sympathomimetic, the patient's vital signs must be monitored. Caution should be used when administering terbutaline to patients with cardiovascular disease or hypertension.

Dosage

The standard dose is two inhalations, 1 minute apart, from a metered-dose inhaler.

Terbutaline can also be administered by subcutaneous injection. The usual dose is 0.25 milligram. This can be repeated in 15 to 30 minutes if needed.

Route

Terbutaline should be administered by inhalation or by subcutaneous injection as described earlier.

How Supplied

Terbutaline is supplied in aerosol canisters. Each spray delivers approximately 0.20 mg of the drug.

Terbutaline for subcutaneous injection is supplied in vials containing 1 milligram of the drug in 1 milliliter of solvent.

Isoetharine (Bronkosol®)

Description

Bronkosol® is a sympathomimetic similar in chemical structure to epinephrine. It exhibits a slight specificity for β_2-adrenergic receptors, thus reducing the potential for cardiac toxicity. Its onset of action is similar to that of epinephrine; however, it has a longer duration of action.

Indications

- Bronchial asthma
- Reversible bronchospasm associated with chronic bronchitis and emphysema

Contraindications

Bronkosol® should not be administered to any patient with a history of hypersensitivity to any of the ingredients.

Precautions

Palpitations, anxiety, nausea, and dizziness are occasionally seen with the administration of Bronkosol®. As with any epinephrine-type compound, the patient's vital signs should be monitored. Caution should be used when administering Bronkosol® to elderly patients with a history of cardiovascular disease or hypertension.

Dosage

There are three major ways to administer Bronkosol®, each with different dosages. They are as follows:

Method of Administration	Usual Dose	Dilution
Hand nebulizer	4 inhalations	Undiluted
Oxygen aerosolization	0.5 milliliter	1:3 w/saline
Intermittent positive-pressure breathing	0.5 milliliter	1:3 w/saline

Routes

Bronkosol® should be administered only by one of the methods listed earlier.

How Supplied

Bronkosol® is supplied in a 2-milliliter unit dose containing a 1% solution.

Metaproterenol (Alupent®)

Description

Metaproterenol is a sympathomimetic that is selective for β_2-adrenergic receptors. It is an effective bronchodilator with a duration of action up to 4 hours.

Indications

- Bronchial asthma
- Reversible bronchospasm associated with chronic bronchitis and emphysema

Contraindications

Metaproterenol should not be used in patients with cardiac arrhythmias or significant tachycardia.

Precautions

Palpitations, anxiety, nausea, and dizziness may be seen following administration of metaproterenol. As with any sympathomimetic, the vital signs must be monitored. Caution should be used when administering metaproterenol to patients with a history of cardiovascular disease or of hypertension. Use of metaproterenol should be avoided in children during the prehospital phase of emergency medical care.

Dosage

Metaproterenol may be administered by metered-dose inhaler. Each spray contains 0.65 milligram of metaproterenol. The usual single dose is two to three inhalations, a minute apart, as needed.

Metaproterenol may also be administered by small-volume nebulizer. The typical adult dose is 0.2 to 0.3 milliliter of metaproterenol diluted in 2.5-milliliters of normal saline. This is typically administered during 5 to 15 minutes.

Route

Metaproterenol should be administered by inhalation only in the emergency setting.

How Supplied

Metaproterenol (Alupent®) is supplied in metered-dose inhalers with each spray delivering 0.65 milligram of the drug.

The solution for nebulization is supplied in single-dose units of 0.4% (0.2 milliliter of Alupent in 2.5 milliliters of saline) and 0.6% (0.3 milliliter of Alupent in 2.5 milliliters of saline).

Albuterol (Proventil®, Ventolin®)

Description

Like the agents metaproterenol and terbutaline, albuterol is a sympatho-mimetic that is selective for β_2-adrenergic receptors. Once administered it causes bronchodilation with a minimal amount of side effects. Albuterol's duration of action is approximately 5 hours.

Indications

- Bronchial asthma
- Reversible bronchospasm associated with chronic bronchitis and emphysema

Contraindications

Albuterol should not be administered to any patient with a known history of hypersensitivity to the drug.

Precautions

Palpitations, anxiety, nausea, and dizziness may be seen following the administration of albuterol. As with any sympathomimetic, the patient's vital signs must be monitored. Caution should be used when administering albuterol to patients with a history of cardiovascular disease or hypertension.

Dosage

Albuterol can be administered by metered-dose inhaler or small-volume nebulizer. A common initial dose is two sprays when using a metered-dose inhaler. Each spray delivers 90 micrograms of albuterol.

When using a small-volume nebulizer the standard adult dose is 2.5 milligrams (0.5 milliliter of a 0.5% solution diluted in 2.5 milliliters of normal saline). This amount is typically delivered during 5 to 15 minutes.

Ventolin® is also available in the Rotohaler® form. A special 200-microgram Rotocap® is placed in the device and inhaled by the patient.

Route

Albuterol should only be administered by inhalation.

How Supplied

Albuterol (Ventolin®) (Proventil®) is supplied in metered dose inhalers that contain approximately three hundred 90-microgram sprays.

The solution for inhalation is supplied in single-patient vials containing 0.5 milliliter of the drug in 2.5 milliliters of normal saline.

Rotocaps for inhalation are supplied in special 200-microgram capsules.

| Aminophylline |

Description

Aminophylline is a bronchodilator that sometimes proves effective in cases in which sympathomimetics have not been effective. Aminophylline achieves its bronchodilation effects via a different mechanism from the sympathomimetics. In addition to bronchodilation, aminophylline has mild diuretic properties, increases the heart rate, the cardiac output, and may precipitate arrhythmias.

Owing to its mild diuretic and inotropic effects, aminophylline is also used in the management of congestive heart failure and pulmonary edema.

In prehospital emergency care, aminophylline is usually given by slow IV infusion. Some systems also carry aminophylline suppositories for use in special situations.

Indications

- Bronchial asthma
- Reversible bronchospasm associated with chronic bronchitis and emphysema
- Congestive heart failure
- Pulmonary edema

Contraindications

Aminophylline should not be administered to any patient with a history of hypersensitivity to the drug.

Precautions

Extreme caution should be used when administering aminophylline to any patient with a history of cardiovascular disease or hypertension. Any patient receiving aminophylline should have a cardiac monitor. One should be alert for any signs of cardiac irritability, especially PVCs and tachycardia. Hypotension can occur following rapid administration.

Aminophylline should not be administered to patients who are on chronic theophylline therapy (Slo-Bid®, Theo-Dur®, and so on) until the amount of drug in the blood has been obtained (theophylline level).

Dosage

Two major regimens are used in administering aminophylline. The first is for use in patients in whom fluid overload or edema does not appear to be present (that is, acute bronchial asthma):

- Place 250 or 500 milligrams in 90 or 80 milliliters of 5% dextrose, respectively. This can be done with a 100-milliliter IV bag or with a Buretrol® or Volutrol®-type administration sets. This is then infused during 20 to 30 minutes. This mechanism of slow infusion tends to reduce the chances of arrhythmias.

In patients with congestive heart failure, or in patients in whom any additional fluid might be dangerous, a more concentrated infusion is prepared:

- Place 250 or 500 milligrams (2 to 5 milligrams per kilogram) in 20 milliliters of 5% dextrose in water. This is then infused during 20 to 30 minutes using a Buretrol or Volutrol-type administration set.

Route

Parenteral aminophylline should only be given by slow IV infusion by one of the regimens discussed earlier.

How Supplied

Aminophylline is supplied in ampules containing 250 milligrams in 10 milliliters of solvent or containing 500 milligrams in 20 milliliters of solvent.

SUMMARY

Respiratory emergencies are a serious and potentially fatal condition if not treated immediately. Prompt recognition of the signs and symptoms of respiratory distress is essential. Oxygen is the primary drug for treating any respiratory problem. Many types of medical problems, especially asthma and anaphylaxis, respond only to the medications discussed in this chapter.

DRUGS USED IN TREATMENT OF METABOLIC-ENDOCRINE EMERGENCIES

INTRODUCTION

Glands that secrete hormones directly into the blood, without the aid of ducts, are called **endocrine glands**. With the exception of the pancreas they rarely cause emergency disorders. Occasionally the thyroid, the endocrine gland that controls metabolic rate, will begin secreting excess thyroid hormones. This disorder, called "thyroid storm," is characterized by increased heart rate, loss of body weight, and congestive heart failure. Fortunately, it is relatively rare and probably would not be diagnosed in the prehospital phase of emergency medical care. Although this chapter is devoted to metabolic-endocrine emergencies, we will primarily discuss the pancreatic disorder diabetes mellitus.

DIABETES MELLITUS

The pancreas is located in the abdominal cavity within the folds of the small intestine. Within the pancreas is an area called the **islets of Langerhans**. The islets of Langerhans has three types of cells that secrete three hormones. The α cells secrete the hormone **glucagon**. The β cells secrete **insulin**. Recently, a third hormone, secreted from the δ cells, called **somatostatin**, has been isolated. Insulin is required for the passage of glucose into the cells. Without insulin the blood glucose level rises. Glucagon

TABLE 8–1   Comparison of Insulin Types

Type	Time of Onset (Hours)	Duration of Action (Hours)
Regular Insulin	1	6
NPH or Lente	2	24
Ultralente	6	36

causes stored carbohydrates, especially glycogen, to be broken down to glucose. When the blood sugar level falls, glucagon is released, which then causes a release of stored carbohydrates. Somatostatin inhibits the secretion of both insulin and glucagon. Functionally, it is similar to growth hormone.

Diabetes mellitus is caused when β cells of the pancreas reduce the amount of insulin secreted. As this occurs, the blood glucose level gets progressively higher. If allowed to progress untreated, the patient will eventually lapse into diabetic coma. Because the signs and symptoms occur early, patients usually seek medical help before coma ensues. Once diagnosed, the patient will most likely be placed on either oral or injectible insulin. If an excessive amount of insulin is taken, or if the patient fails to eat properly, then **hypoglycemia** can develop.

There are three major classifications of injectible insulin. **Regular insulin** is classified as fast acting. **Lente** or **NPH** insulin is classified as intermediate acting. Long-lasting insulin is called **ultralente**. Table 8–1 helps illustrate the relationship between the three classes.

In this chapter we will discuss **insulin, glucagon, 50% dextrose in water (D$_{50}$W), glucola,** and **thiamine.** All of these agents, except thiamine, are primarily used in the management of the diabetic patient. Thiamine should be administered before D$_{50}$W to any patient with coma of an unknown origin, especially if alcoholism is suspected.

Insulin

Description

Insulin is a protein secreted by the β cells of the islets of Langerhans. It is responsible for promoting the uptake of glucose by the cells. In diabetics, where insulin secretion has diminished, supplemental insulin must be obtained by injection.

A blood glucose approximation should be obtained in all diabetic emergencies. Every EMS unit carrying insulin and 50% dextrose should also carry Dextrostix® reagent strips for approximating blood glucose levels. Based on the results of the Dextrostix®, in conjunction with the physical examination, the differential diagnosis between hypoglycemia and ketoacidosis can usually be made. If there is any doubt about the etiology of diabetic coma, glucose should be administered.

Indication

- Diabetic ketoacidosis

Contraindications

Insulin should be administered only when ketoacidosis has been confirmed. Insulin is almost always administered in the emergency department and not during the prehospital phase of emergency medical care.

Precautions

Repeated measurements of the blood glucose, including possible administration of glucose, are necessary.

Dosage

A standard dose for diabetic coma is 10 to 25 units regular insulin IV followed by an infusion at 0.1 unit per kilogram per hour.

Route

In an emergency setting, insulin should be given intravenously or intramuscularly.

How Supplied

Insulin injection is supplied in 10-milliliter vials containing 100 units per milliliter.

> ### Glucagon

Description

Glucagon is a protein secreted by the α cells of the pancreas. When released it causes a breakdown of stored glycogen to glucose. It also inhibits the synthesis of glycogen from glucose. Both actions tend to cause an increase in circulating blood glucose. In hypoglycemia the administration of glucagon increases blood glucose levels. The drug of choice in the management of insulin-induced hypoglycemia is still $D_{50}W$. A return to consciousness is seen almost immediately following the administration of glucose. A return to consciousness following the administration of glucagon usually takes from 5 to 20 minutes. Glucagon is only effective if there are sufficient stores of glycogen in the liver.

Glucagon exerts a positive inotropic action on the heart and decreases renal vascular resistance.

Indication

- Hypoglycemia

Contraindications

Because glucagon is a protein, hypersensitivity may occur.

Precautions

Glucagon is only effective if there are sufficient stores of glycogen within the liver. In an emergency situation, intravenous glucose is the agent of choice.

Glucagon should be administered with caution to patients with a history of cardiovascular or renal disease.

Dosage

A standard initial dose is 0.5 to 1.0 units intravenously.

Route

Glucagon can be administered intravenously, intramuscularly, or sub-cutaneously.

How Supplied

Glucagon must be reconstituted before administration. It is supplied in rubber-stoppered vials containing 1 unit of powder and 1 milliliter of diluting solution. It must be used or refrigerated after reconstitution.

$D_{50}W$

Description

"Dextrose" is used to describe the six-carbon sugar **d-glucose**, which is the principal form of carbohydrate used by the body. In hypoglycemia, the rapid administration of glucose is essential. When the hypoglycemic patient is comatose, glucose cannot be given by mouth and should be given as IV $D_{50}W$ solution.

Indications

- Hypoglycemia
- Coma of unknown origin

Contraindications

There are no major contraindications to the IV administration of $D_{50}W$ to a patient with suspected hypoglycemia. Even if a patient was suffering from ketoacidosis, the amount of glucose present in 50 milliliters of 50% dextrose would not adversely affect the clinical outcome.

Precautions

It is important to perform a Dextrostix and draw a sample of blood before initiating an IV infusion and giving 50% dextrose. Localized venous irritation may occur when smaller veins are used. Infiltration of 50% dextrose may result in tissue necrosis.

Dosage

The standard dosage of 50% dextrose in hypoglycemia is 25 grams (50 milliliters of a 50% solution) intravenously. If an initial dose is ineffective, a second dose of 25 grams can also be given.

Route

Fifty percent dextrose is only given intravenously. Concentrated glucose solutions can cause venous irritation if administered for an extended period.

How Supplied

Fifty percent dextrose is supplied in prefilled syringes containing 25 grams of d-glucose in 50 milliliters of water.

Glucola

Description

Glucola is a carbonated, cola-flavored carbohydrate solution. It is useful in the management of hypoglycemic patients who are conscious. It is approximately 30% glucose and also contains several other simple and complex carbohydrates.

Indication

- Conscious patients with suspected hypoglycemia

Contraindications

Glucola should not be given to any semiconscious or unconscious patient. It also should not be used in patients who appear nauseated. In these cases IV 50% dextrose is indicated.

Precautions

When giving glucola, it is important to assure that the airway is patent (open).

Dosage

Glucola should be slowly sipped by the patient until a feeling of improvement is reported. It is not essential to administer the entire bottle.

Route

Glucola should only be taken by mouth.

How Supplied

Glucola is supplied in 300-milliliter bottles.

Thiamine

Description

Thiamine is an important vitamin commonly referred to as vitamin B_1. A vitamin is a substance that the body cannot manufacture but that is required for metabolism. Most of the vitamins required by the body are obtained through the diet. Thiamine is required for the conversion of pyruvic acid to acetyl-coenzyme-A. Without this step a significant amount of the energy available in glucose cannot be obtained. The brain is extremely sensitive to thiamine deficiency.

Chronic alcohol intake interferes with the absorption, intake, and use of thiamine. A significant percentage of alcoholics have thiamine deficiency. During extended periods of fasting, neurological symptoms owing to thiamine deficiency can occur. Any comatose patients, especially those who are suspected to be alcoholic, should receive IV thiamine in addition to the administration of 50% dextrose or Narcan.

Indications

- Coma of unknown origin, especially if alcohol may be involved
- Delerium tremens

Contraindications

There are no contraindications to the administration of thiamine in the emergency setting.

Precautions

A few cases of hypersensitivity to thiamine have been reported.

Dosage

The emergency dose of thiamine is 100 milligrams intravenously or intramuscularly.

Route

Thiamine can be given either intravenously or intramuscularly. The intravenous route is preferred in emergency medicine.

How Supplied

Thiamine is supplied in 1-milliliter ampules containing 100 milligrams of the vitamin.

SUMMARY

Diabetes mellitus is probably the most common metabolic-endocrine emergency seen in the prehospital phase of emergency medical care. Hypoglycemia, if not immediately treated, can result in serious and permanent brain damage. It is important to remember that acute metabolic-endocrine disorders can cause a wide range of signs and symptoms from bizarre behavior to coma. Administration of 50% dextrose and thiamine to all patients with coma of unknown etiology may prevent neurological sequelae and may elucidate the etiology of the coma.

DRUGS USED IN TREATMENT OF NEUROLOGICAL EMERGENCIES

INTRODUCTION

Emergencies involving the nervous system can be devastating. In addition, they are also notoriously difficult to manage. Signs and symptoms of neurological disorders can range from slight headache to coma. They may be temporary or permanent. Prompt recognition and treatment is essential.

NEUROLOGICAL TRAUMA

Head injuries are an all too common result of automobile and motorcycle accidents. Although encased within the protective skull, the brain is quite susceptible to injury. Following craniocerebral trauma, cerebral edema occurs within 24 hours.

The primary treatment of patients with blunt or penetrating head injury is supportive. Airway management is of paramount importance, and continuous monitoring of blood pressure to detect occult blood loss in major trauma is mandatory. Pharmacological agents that have proved effective in the management of neurological emergencies include **dexamethasone**, which is thought to be of use in reducing brain edema, and **mannitol**, an osmotic diuretic that is also useful in reducing brain edema and is faster-acting than dexamethasone.

The management of spinal cord injuries is principally supportive. The severity of the injury will depend on the anatomical location of the spinal cord damage. Sometimes, following injury to the spinal cord, shock will occur (neurogenic shock). In these cases the body loses control over peripheral vascular tone. Vasopressor agents, such as norepinephrine, are indicated to assure maintenance of blood pressure.

The drugs on the following pages are frequently used in the prehospital phase of emergency medical care in the management of traumatic neurological emergencies.

Dexamethasone (Decadron®, Hexadrol®)

Description

The role of steroids in the management of cerebral edema remains controversial. The mechanism and extent to which dexamethasone decreases cerebral edema, if indeed it does, is unclear.

Dexamethasone is a synthetic steroid chemically related to the natural hormones secreted by the adrenal cortex. Decadron is classified as a long-acting steroid with a plasma half-life of about 5 hours. In general medical practice, steroids have a wide range of uses. Effective as anti-inflammatory agents, they are used in the management of allergic reactions and occasionally as an adjunctive agent in the management of shock.

It is generally agreed that a large single dose of steroids has little harmful effects. Consequently, it is used frequently in patients with cerebral edema, both in the emergency department and in the prehospital setting.

Indications

- Cerebral edema
- Possibly effective as an adjunctive agent in the management of shock

Contraindications

There are no major contraindications to the use of dexamethasone in the acute management of cerebral edema.

Precautions

A single dose of dexamethasone is all that should be given in the prehospital phase of care. Long-term steroid therapy can cause gastrointestinal bleeding, prolonged wound healing, and suppression of adrenocortical steroids.

Dosage

The dose of dexamethasone varies considerably from physician to physician. The usual range is 4 to 24 milligrams with 12 milligrams intravenously being a commonly used dose. High-dose Decadron® therapy, however, with up to 100 milligrams of the drug, is sometimes given.

Route

Dexamethasone is administered intravenously for treatment of acute cerebral edema.

How Supplied

Decadron® is supplied in two concentrations. The most common is the 4 milligrams per milliliter. It is supplied in prefilled syringes containing 1 milliliter of the drug and in vials containing 5 milligrams.

A second concentration, containing 24 milligrams per milliliter, is also available. It is supplied in 5- and 10-milliliter ampules. This concentration should only be used intravenously.

Mannitol (Osmotrol®)

Description

Mannitol is a six-carbon sugar compound that has osmotic diuretic properties. Mannitol promotes movement of fluid from the intracellular into the extracellular space. Because it dehydrates brain tissue, mannitol has proven effective in the management of cerebral edema and reduces intracranial pressure.

Indications

- Acute cerebral edema
- Blood transfusion reactions

Contraindications

Mannitol should not be used in any patient with acute pulmonary edema or severe pulmonary congestion. It should not be used in any patient who is profoundly hypovolemic.

Precautions

Rapid administration of mannitol can cause a transitory increase in intravascular volume and can result in congestive heart failure. The diuresis that accompanies mannitol therapy can cause sodium depletion.

One problem in the use of mannitol in the prehospital phase of emergency medical care is crystallization of the drug. The more concentrated the solution, the more tendency it has to crystallize at low temperatures. Crystallization begins as temperatures approach 45°F. Anytime a concentrated solution of mannitol is used, usually 15% or greater, an in-line filter should be present. It is important to remember that microscopic crystals appear long before those that can be seen to the naked eye.

If mannitol solution does crystallize, it should be warmed slowly in boiling water until the crystals disappear. It should be removed from EMS vehicles that are not parked in heated areas during colder weather.

Dosage

Administer 500 milliliters of a 20% solution by IV infusion over 30 to 60 minutes.

The slower rate of infusion helps eliminate the chances of inducing circulatory overload and congestive heart failure.

Route

Mannitol should be given intravenously.

How Supplied

Mannitol is supplied in 250 and 500 milliliters of a 20% solution for IV infusion. A 25% solution in 50 milliliters is available for slow IV bolus.

NONTRAUMATIC NEUROLOGICAL EMERGENCIES

There are many acute nontraumatic neurological disorders. Drugs, poisonings, and metabolic derangements can precipitate neurological emergencies. There is little that can be done for stroke and brain tumors in the prehospital phase of emergency medical care. Seizures attributable to epilepsy and other disorders can be managed in the field, however.

Seizures are one of the most frequently encountered neurological emergencies. One seizure followed by another seizure, without an intervening period of consciousness, is called **status epilepticus**, and constitutes a serious threat to life. Status epilepticus should be terminated as quickly as possible.

The most common drug used to terminate seizure activity is IV diazepam (Valium®). Phenytoin (Dilantin®) and phenobarbital are also effective, however. In the following section of this chapter these three drugs and their roles in prehospital care are discussed.

Diazepam (Valium®)

Description

Valium®, one of the most frequently prescribed medications in the United States, is used in the management of anxiety and stress. Valium® is effective in treating the tremors and anxiety associated with alcohol withdrawal. It is also an effective skeletal muscle relaxant, which makes it an effective adjunct in orthopedic injuries. It is a good premedication for minor operative procedures and cardioversion because it induces amnesia, which diminishes the patient's recall of such procedures.

In emergency medicine Valium® is principally used for its anticonvulsant properties. It suppresses the spread of seizure activity through the motor cortex of the brain. It does not appear to abolish the abnormal discharge focus, however.

Indications

- Major motor seizures
- Status epilepticus
- Premedication before cardioversion
- Skeletal muscle relaxant
- Acute anxiety states

Contraindications

Valium® should not be administered to any patient with a history of hypersensitivity to the drug.

Precautions

Because Valium® is a relatively short-acting drug, seizure activity may recur. In such cases, an additional dose may be required.

Injectible Valium® can cause local venous irritation. To minimize this, it should only be injected into relatively large veins and should not be given faster than 1 milliliter per minute.

Valium® is incompatible with many medications. Any time Valium® is given intravenously in conjunction with other drugs, the IV line should be adequately flushed.

Dosage

In the management of seizures, the usual dose of Valium® is 5 to 10 milligrams IV. In many instances it may be necessary to give Valium® directly into the vein as the seizure activity will prevent the insertion of an indwelling catheter. When given directly into a vein, it is essential that a large vein, preferably in the antecubital fossa, is used.

In acute anxiety reactions, the standard dosage is 2 to 5 milligrams intramuscularly versus intravenously.

To induce amnesia during cardioversion, a dosage of 5 to 15 milligrams of Valium® is given intravenously. Peak effects are seen in 5 to 10 minutes.

Routes

For the treatment of seizures, Valium® should be given intravenously by slow IV push. It can be injected intramuscularly, but absorption via this route is variable. When an IV line cannot be started, parenteral diazepam can be administered rectally with a similar onset of action.

How Supplied

Valium® is supplied in ampules and prefilled syringes containing 10 milligrams in 2 milliliters of solvent.

Phenytoin (Dilantin®)

Description

Phenytoin is an effective anticonvulsant. Its onset of action, however, is considerably longer than for Valium®. In most emergency situations the seizure should be first controlled with Valium®. If seizure activity recurs, phenytoin can be administered.

Phenytoin also is used to treat arrhythmias caused by digitalis toxicity. This use of the drug is discussed in Chapter 6.

Indications

- Major motor seizures
- Status epilepticus
- Arrhythmias owing to digitalis toxicity

Contraindications

Phenytoin should not be given to any patient with a history of hypersensitivity to the drug.

Precautions

Phenytoin should not be administered with 5% dextrose in water as precipitation may occur.

Careful monitoring of blood pressure should be made following IV administration of phenytoin as hypotension has been known to occur. Venous irritation can occur because of the alkalinity of the solution.

Dosage

The loading dose of phenytoin is typically 10 to 15 milligrams per kilogram. This should be administered no faster than 50 milligrams per minute. Phenytoin should be diluted with normal saline as dilution with 5% dextrose may result in precipitation of the drug.

Route

In emergency medicine, phenytoin should be administered intravenously only.

How Supplied

Dilantin® is supplied in 2- and 5-milliliter ampules containing 50 milligrams per milliliter. A 2-milliliter prefilled syringe is also available.

Phenobarbital

Description

Phenobarbital belongs to a class of drugs called **barbiturates**. Barbiturates have many uses in medicine. They are central nervous system depressants and are used in the management of insomnia, anxiety, and as anticonvulsants.

Phenobarbital is an effective anticonvulsant of relatively low toxicity.

Indications

- Major motor seizures
- Status epilepticus
- Acute anxiety states

Contraindications

Phenobarbital should not be administered to any patient with a history of hypersensitivity to the barbiturates.

Precautions

Respiratory depression and hypotension can occur following IV administration of phenobarbital. Constant monitoring of respiratory pattern and blood pressure is essential. Administration of phenobarbital to children may result in hyperactive behavior.

Dosage

The standard dosage of phenobarbital in the management of status epilepticus is 100 to 250 milligrams intravenously given slowly.

How Supplied

Phenobarbital is supplied in 1-milliliter ampules containing 130 milligrams of the drug. The solution may be diluted with 9 milliliters of 5% dextrose in water to give a concentration of 13 milligrams per milliliter. This dilution facilitates slow and constant intravenous administration.

SUMMARY

In the management of acute head injury, dexamethasone and mannitol have proved effective in reducing cerebral edema. It is important to remember that stabilization of the cervical spine, maintenance of the airway, and supplemental delivery of oxygen are of primary importance.

In a general motor seizure, as occasionally occurs, the primary treatment is that of protecting the patient from injury. It is important to remember that most epileptic patients are already taking orally one or two anticonvulsant medications. The judicious use of the parenteral agents discussed in this chapter is therefore indicated. It is helpful to the emergency physician to obtain blood samples from seizure patients prior to the administration of an anticonvulsant. Some authorities believe that a significant percentage of patients present with general motor seizures because of little or no patient drug compliance. Blood studies taken before the administration of anticonvulsants will aid the physician in making a diagnosis.

10

DRUGS USED IN MANAGEMENT OF OBSTETRICAL AND GYNECOLOGICAL EMERGENCIES

INTRODUCTION

Prehospital care for most obstetrical and gynecological emergencies is supportive. There are two complications, however, that necessitate intervention with pharmacological agents. These are toxemia of pregnancy and severe vaginal bleeding. **Magnesium sulfate** has proved effective in controlling the convulsions associated with toxemia of pregnancy. **Pitocin®**, a drug chemically identical to the hormone oxytocin, is effective in causing uterine contraction and will control many cases of postpartum vaginal bleeding.

SEVERE VAGINAL BLEEDING

Vaginal bleeding that occurs during the first trimester of pregnancy is usually owing to spontaneous abortion or ectopic pregnancy. During the third trimester of pregnancy, vaginal bleeding is most frequently caused by either abruptio placenta or placenta previa.

Bleeding following childbirth is common. Hypovolemic shock can develop when blood loss is in excess of 500 milliliters. Severe vaginal bleeding can be a life-threatening emergency, necessitating immediate therapy.

The management of severe vaginal bleeding is similar to that employed with any other types of severe hemorrhage. Initial treatment should include airway maintenance, administration of supplemental oxygen, and infusion of intravenous volume expanders. In addition, the IV administration of Pitocin® in postpartum hemorrhage can be effective in controlling severe vaginal bleeding.

Oxytocin (Pitocin®)

Description

Oxytocin is a naturally occurring hormone that is secreted by the posterior pituitary. It causes contraction of uterine smooth muscle and lactation.

Oxytocin is used to induce labor in selected cases and is also effective in inducing uterine contractions following delivery, thereby controlling postpartum hemorrhage.

When a baby is placed on the breast, the sucking action causes the posterior pituitary to release oxytocin. It is important to remember this inherent mechanism whenever confronted by a patient suffering moderate to severe postpartum bleeding.

Indication

- Postpartum hemorrhage

Contraindications

In the prehospital setting, oxytocin should be administered only to patients suffering severe postpartum bleeding. Before administration it is essential to verify that the baby has been delivered and that there is not an additional fetus in the uterus.

Precautions

Excess oxytocin can cause overstimulation of the uterus and possible rupture. Hypertension, cardiac arrhythmia, and anaphylaxis have been reported in conjunction with the administration of oxytocin. Vital signs and uterine tone should be monitored.

Dosage

The following are two regimens for the administration of oxytocin in the management of patients with postpartum hemorrhage:

- 3 to 10 units can be administered intramuscularly following delivery of the placenta.

- 10 to 20 units can be placed in either 500 or 1000 milliliters of D_5W or lactated Ringer's. This should be titrated according to the severity of the bleeding and the uterine response.

Routes

Oxytocin should only be administered intramuscularly or by slow IV infusion.

How Supplied

Pitocin is supplied in 0.5- and 1-milliliter ampules containing 10 milligrams per milliliter. A 1-milliliter prefilled syringe containing the same concentration is also available.

TOXEMIA OF PREGNANCY

Toxemia of pregnancy occurs in approximately 4 percent of all pregnancies. The early stage is called **preeclampsia** and is characterized by severe headache, malaise, generalized body edema, and significantly elevated blood pressure. It is not uncommon to see systolic values over 200 millimeters of mercury and diastolic values over 100 millimeters of mercury. Preeclampsia can progress to convulsions, coma, and death. This stage, called **eclampsia**, is often fatal.

Eclampsia must be treated vigorously. **Magnesium sulfate** is the drug of choice for controlling convulsions associated with toxemia. In addition, it may be necessary to administer an antihypertensive agent, such as those discussed in Chapter 6, to prevent the complications of hypertensive crisis. The decision to administer an antihypertensive in the prehospital phase of emergency medical care rests with the base station physician. Each case should be treated individually.

Magnesium Sulfate

Description

Magnesium sulfate is a central nervous system depressant effective in the management of seizures associated with toxemia of pregnancy. It is used for the initial therapy of convulsions. After cessation of seizure activity, other anticonvulsant agents may be administered.

Indication

- Eclampsia (seizures accompanying pregnancy)

Contraindications

Magnesium sulfate should not be administered to any patient with heart block or recent myocardial infarction.

Precautions

Magnesium sulfate, like other central nervous system depressants, can cause hypotension, circulatory collapse, and depression of cardiac and respiratory function. The most immediate danger is respiratory depression. Calcium chloride should be readily available for IV administration as an antidote in case respiratory depression occurs.

Dosage

The standard dosage for the management of convulsions associated with toxemia of pregnancy is 1 gram intravenously.

Route

In the setting of toxemia, magnesium sulfate should only be administered intravenously.

How Supplied

Magnesium sulfate is supplied in prefilled syringes containing 5 and 10 milliliters of a 50% solution.

SUMMARY

Most obstetrical and gynecological emergencies are not managed in the field. Prehospital treatment should include stabilization of the airway, administration of supplemental oxygen, and replacement of intravascular volume. In severe postpartum bleeding the administration of Pitocin is often effective. In toxemia of pregnancy, magnesium sulfate may be used during the prehospital phase of emergency medical care to control convulsions. The definitive treatment of toxemia of pregnancy is delivery of the fetus.

11

DRUGS USED IN MANAGEMENT OF TOXICOLOGICAL EMERGENCIES

INTRODUCTION

The following discussion of prehospital drugs used in the management of toxicological emergencies is divided into three general categories:

Anaphylaxis

- Epinephrine
- Diphenhydramine (Benadryl®)
- Methylprednisolone (Solu-Medrol®)
- Hydrocortisone (Solu-Cortef®)

Poisonings

- Syrup of ipecac
- Activated charcoal
- Atropine sulfate
- Pralidoxime (Protopam®)
- Amyl nitrite

Overdoses

- Naloxone ((Narcan®)
- Physostigmine (Antilirium®)

ANAPHYLAXIS

In severe allergic reactions, or anaphylaxis, as it is more commonly called, excess release of histamine and other substances can cause severe bronchospasm, dilation of the peripheral blood vessels, and loss of fluid into the tissue spaces. Clinically, anaphylaxis is characterized by restlessness, wheezing, dyspnea, increased heart rate, and diminished blood pressure. If untreated, laryngeal edema, laryngospasm, and respiratory failure can rapidly develop.

Treatment of anaphylaxis is aimed at immediate alleviation of bronchospasm by sympathomimetics. Sustained actions are obtained with the use of a potent antihistamine and, frequently, steroids.

Epinephrine

Description

The primary drug used in the management of anaphylaxis is epinephrine. Epinephrine acts on both α- and β-adrenergic receptors. Epinephrine causes immediate bronchodilatation, an increase in the heart rate, and an increase in the force of the cardiac contraction. The therapeutic effects of a subcutaneous dose of epinephrine last only 5 to 15 minutes. Occasionally, it may be necessary to establish an epinephrine infusion to maintain blood pressure and bronchodilation until the effects of the antihistamine and steroids are seen.

Indications

- Anaphylaxis
- Bronchial asthma

Contraindications

When used in the management of life-threatening anaphylaxis, there are no major contraindications to the use of epinephrine.

Precautions

Epinephrine should be protected from light and can be deactivated by alkaline solutions. Any patient receiving epinephrine should be carefully monitored for changes in blood pressure, pulse, and EKG. Palpitations, anxiety, and headache are fairly common complications.

Dosage

In severe anaphylactic shock, IV administration of epinephrine may be required. When given intravenously, the 1:10,000 dilution should be used only. The standard dosage is 0.3 to 0.5 milligrams (3 to 5 milliliters).

In most cases of anaphylaxis, a subcutaneous dose may be adequate. In these cases, the 1:1000 dilution should be used. The dosage ranges from 0.3 to 0.5 milligrams (0.3 to 0.5 milliliters).

In severe and prolonged anaphylactic reactions an IV infusion of epinephrine may be required. The standard method for preparing an epinephrine infusion is to place 2 milligrams of epinephrine 1:1000 in 500 milliliters of D_5W. This gives a concentration of 4 micrograms per milliliter. This should then be administered slowly so as not to exceed 4 micrograms per minute. It is essential to avoid IV infiltration.

Routes

Epinephrine may be given subcutaneously and intravenously as discussed earlier. In severe anaphylaxis, when an IV line cannot be established, epinephrine can be administered transtracheally.

How Supplied

Epinephrine 1:10,000 is supplied in prefilled syringes containing 1 milligram of the drug in 10 milliliters of solvent.

Epinephrine 1:1000 is supplied in ampules and prefilled syringes containing 1 milligram of the drug in 1 milliliter of solvent.

Diphenhydramine (Benadryl®)

Description

When released into the circulation following an allergic reaction, histamine acts on two different receptors. The first type of receptor, called H_1, when stimulated, causes bronchoconstriction and contraction of the gut. The second type of receptor, called H_2, when stimulated, causes peripheral vasodilation and secretion of gastric acids.

Antihistamines are administered after epinephrine in the treatment of anaphylaxis. Epinephrine causes immediate bronchodilation by activating β_2 adrenergic receptors, whereas diphenhydramine inhibits histamine release.

Diphenhydramine is also useful in the treatment of dystonic reactions accompanying phenothiazine use. A dystonic, or extrapyramidal, reaction is characterized by an unusual posture, change in muscle tone, drooling, or uncontrolled movements. It is occasionally seen following the administration of antipsychotic medications (Haldol®, Thorazine®, Mellaril®) as well as certain medications used for nausea and vomiting (Phenergan®, Compazine®). Diphenhydramine, when administered, causes marked improvement, if not total resolution of the symptoms.

Indications

- Anaphylaxis
- Allergic reactions
- Dystonic (extrapyramidal) reactions

Contraindications

Diphenhydramine should not be used in the management of lower respiratory diseases such as asthma.

Precautions

Hypotension, headache, palpitations, and tachycardia have been known to occur following administration of diphenhydramine. Sedation, drowsiness, and disturbed coordination are also common.

Dosage

The standard dosage of diphenhydramine is 25 to 50 milligrams, either intravenously or intramuscularly.

Routes

Diphenhydramine should be administered intravenously or intramuscularly.

How Supplied

Diphenhydramine is supplied in ampules and prefilled syringes containing 50 milligrams of the drug in 1 milliliter of solvent.

Methylprednisolone (Solu-Medrol®)

Description

Methylprednisolone is a synthetic steroid with potent anti-inflammatory properties. The pharmacological actions of the steroids are vast and complex. The discussion of the pharmacological actions is not within the scope of this text. Methylprednisolone is considered an intermediate-acting steroid with a plasma half-life of about 3 to 4 hours. Like the other adrenocorticosteroids, it is effective as an adjunct in the management of severe anaphylaxis.

Indications

- Severe anaphylaxis
- Possibly effective as an adjunctive agent in the management of shock

Contraindications

There are no major contraindications to the use of methylprednisolone in the acute management of severe anaphylaxis.

Precautions

Methylprednisolone is supplied in powder form that must be reconstituted in the supplied Mix-O-Vial® system. Once reconstituted, it should be used within 48 hours.

Dosage

The standard dosage of methylprednisolone in the management of severe anaphylaxis is 125 to 250 milligrams intravenously.

Route

Methylprednisolone may be administered intravenously or intramuscularly. The intravenous route is preferred in emergency medicine.

How Supplied

Methylprednisolone is supplied in Mix-O-Vials containing 125 milligrams of the drug.

Hydrocortisone (Solu-Cortef®)

Description

Hydrocortisone is a potent anti-inflammatory agent. The pharmacological actions of the steroids are vast and complex. The discussion of these actions is not within the scope of this text. Hydrocortisone is considered a short-acting steroid with a plasma half-life of 90 minutes. Like the other adrenocorticosteroids, it is effective as an adjunct in the management of severe anaphylaxis.

Indications

- Severe anaphylaxis
- Possibly effective as an adjunctive agent in the management of shock

Contraindications

There are no major contraindications to the use of hydrocortisone in the acute management of anaphylaxis.

Precautions

Hydrocortisone is supplied in powder form that must be reconstituted in the supplied Mix-O-Vial system. Once reconstituted it should be used within 48 hours.

Dosage

The standard dosage of hydrocortisone in the management of severe anaphylaxis is 100 to 250 milligrams intravenously.

Route

The IV route is preferred in emergency medicine.

How Supplied

Hydrocortisone is supplied in Mix-O-Vials containing 100 and 250 milligrams of the drug.

POISONING

The term **poisoning** is used to describe the accidental or inadvertent ingestion of a substance that causes a destructive effect on the body. **Overdose**, although actually a form of poisoning, is used to describe the intentional ingestion of a substance by a patient during an attempt at self-destruction. In this discussion of toxicological emergencies, overdose and poisoning will be addressed separately.

The first step in the management of any poisoning is to locate and identify the poison. Although this is not always possible, when known it can aid in definitive treatment of the patient. Treatment of the patient is divided into two stages. The first stage is to prevent or reduce absorption of the toxin into the body. This can be done by inducing vomiting in conscious patients. Vomiting is effectively induced by the drug **syrup of ipecac**. **Activated charcoal** is a common and effective adsorbent.

If indicated, the second phase of management involves the administration of an **antidote**. Antidotes are drugs that tend to counteract the toxic effects of a poison. Usually, prehospital administration of antidotes is not indicated, but **organophosphate** or **cyanide** poisonings require prehospital administration of antidotes. **Atropine sulfate** and **pralidoxime** (2-PAM) can be effective in the management of organophosphate poisonings. **Amyl nitrite** is of use in reversing some of the toxic effects associated with cyanide poisoning.

Syrup of Ipecac

Description

Syrup of ipecac is a potent and effective emetic. It acts as a local irritant on the enteric tract and on emetic centers within the brain, thus causing emesis. To assure complete evacuation of the stomach, the administration of ipecac is usually followed by several glasses of warm water. Recently, some studies have advocated the use of carbonated beverages instead of warm water. Carbonated beverages may cause emesis sooner. Emesis, following administration, usually occurs within 5 to 10 minutes.

Indications

- Poisoning
- Overdose

Contraindications

Vomiting should not be induced in any patient with impaired consciousness. It should also not be induced when the ingested substance is a strong acid base (that is, caustic ingestion) or petroleum distillate.

In addition, administration of syrup of ipecac is not indicated when the ingested agent was an antiemetic, especially of the phenothiazine type.

The trend in the management of toxicological emergencies has been to use activated charcoal alone without ipecac. This is primarily because of the increased risk of aspiration associated with ipecac usage.

Precautions

It is important to monitor constantly the patient's airway during and following emesis. Activated charcoal should only be administered after vomiting has occurred.

Dosage

The standard dose of syrup of ipecac is 15 to 30 milliliters orally followed by several glasses of warm water or carbonated soda.

Route

Syrup of ipecac should only be administered orally.

How Supplied

Syrup of ipecac is supplied in bottles containing 1 ounce (approximately 30 milliliters).

Activated Charcoal

Description

Activated charcoal is a fine black powder that binds and adsorbs ingested toxins still present in the gastrointestinal tract following emesis. Once bound to the activated charcoal, the combined complex is excreted from the body.

Indication

- Poisoning (following emesis, or in cases in which emesis may be contraindicated)

Contraindications

There are no major contraindications to the use of activated charcoal in severe poisoning.

Precautions

Activated charcoal should not be administered to the patient who has an altered level of consciousness unless administered by nasogastric tube and the airway protected by an endotracheal tube. If emesis is to be induced with ipecac, it is often best to wait until the patient has vomited to administer activated charcoal.

Dosage

The standard dosage in the management of poisoning is 2 tablespoons (50 grams) mixed with a glass of water. This is then administered orally or through a nasogastric tube.

Route

Activated charcoal should only be administered orally in a slurry solution made with water as described earlier.

How Supplied

Activated charcoal is supplied in bottles containing 25 grams of the drug.

ORGANOPHOSPHATE POISONINGS

Organophosphates serve as the active agents in many insecticides and nerve gases. Common insecticide preparations that employ organophosphates include Parathion®, Malathion®, and EPN. These insecticides are widely used in agriculture and are occasionally found within the home. They are easily absorbed through the skin, lungs, and by ingestion. Patients suspected of suffering organophosphate poisoning should have their clothes removed immediately to prevent continued absorption. Organophosphates deactivate, by phosphorylation, the enzyme cholinesterase. Cholinesterase is vital to normal body function as it deactivates the neurotransmitter acetylcholine. Acetylcholine is the neurotransmitter used by both the voluntary and the parasympathetic nervous system.

Signs and symptoms of organophosphate poisoning include ocular pain, watery nasal discharge, diaphoresis, bradycardia, abdominal cramps, and vomiting. Advanced organophosphate poisoning is characterized by involuntary muscle twitching, generalized weakness, paralysis, and respiratory depression.

In the advanced stage, the prompt administration of atropine and possibly 2-PAM is essential. Atropine binds to acetylcholine receptors, thus diminishing the actions of acetylcholine. Cholinesterase is reactivated by 2-PAM.

Atropine Sulfate

Description

Atropine sulfate is a potent parasympatholytic. It blocks acetylcholine receptors, thus aiding the management of organophosphate poisonings. Organophosphate poisonings inhibit the enzyme cholinesterase. Often, large doses are required to achieve atropinization. Severe poisonings, especially those characterized by paralysis and muscle twitching, require pralidoxime (2-PAM), in addition to atropine.

Indications

- Organophosphate poisoning
- Bradycardias that are hemodynamically significant

Contraindications

There are no contraindications to atropine when used in the management of severe organophosphate poisoning.

Precautions

It is important to remove all clothing from a patient who has suffered organophosphate poisoning. The patient must then be completely bathed to remove all residual organophosphate present on the skin.

Dosage

One milligram of atropine should be administered initially to determine whether or not the patient is tolerant to atropine. If the patient responds to the diagnostic dose, then most likely he or she is not severely poisoned or is not tolerant to atropine. If there is no improvement, a second dose of 2 to 5 milligrams may be indicated for an adult (0.05 milligrams per kilogram for a child). Doses exceeding 100 milligrams are sometimes required to treat severe organophosphate poisoning. In prehospital care, following the initial administration of atropine, prompt transportation to an emergency department is indicated.

Route

In severe organophosphate poisoning, atropine sulfate is administered intravenously.

How Supplied

Atropine sulfate is supplied in prefilled syringes containing 1 milligram of the drug in 10 milliliters of solvent.

Pralidoxime (2-PAM) (Protopam®)

Description

Pralidoxime is a cholinesterase reactivator. It chemically removes the phosphate group from cholinesterase that was transferred from an organophosphate poison. Once cholinesterase is reactivated, it can deactivate acetylcholine. Pralidoxime also detoxifies some organophosphates by direct chemical reaction.

Pralidoxime should be reserved for severe organophosphate poisonings characterized by muscle twitching and paralysis. It should follow atropinization.

Indication

- Severe organophosphate poisoning

Contraindications

Pralidoxime should not be used in cases of poisoning resulting from inorganic phosphates or the carbamate class of insecticides.

Precautions

Always protect yourself and other rescuers when caring for the victim of organophosphate poisoning.

Intravenous administration should be carried out slowly as tachycardia, laryngospasm, and muscle rigidity have been seen with rapid administration. When used in conjunction with atropine, the effects of atropinization may be seen much earlier than expected. This is especially true if the atropine dose has been large. Excitement and manic behavior have been known to occur immediately following recovery from unconsciousness in a few cases.

Dosage

One gram of pralidoxime should be placed in 250 to 500 milliliters of normal saline and infused over 30 minutes.

Route

Pralidoxime should be administered by IV infusion or slow IV bolus only.

How Supplied

Pralidoxime is supplied in 20-milliliter vials with 1 gram of the drug. The drug must be reconstituted with 20 milliliters of sterile water, which is supplied.

CYANIDE POISONING

Cyanide is one of the most rapidly acting and deadly poisons known to humans. It has been used in executions, in the mass suicides in Guyana, and was responsible for several deaths after it was placed into capsules of a popular over-the-counter analgesic.

Cyanide reacts with iron, thus inhibiting cellular respiration, causing cellular hypoxia, and finally death. Clinically, the patient with cyanide poisoning exhibits a rapid respiratory rate, severe headache and, finally, convulsions and death. Cyanide poisoning may produce the peculiar smell of "bitter almonds" on the patient's breath. Treatment, if it is to be effective, must be initiated *immediately*. Amyl nitrite, administered by inhalation, causes hemoglobin to be converted to methemoglobin. Methemoglobin reacts with the toxic cyanide ion to form cyanomethemoglobin, which is enzymatically degraded.

Amyl Nitrite

Description

Amyl nitrite, which is chemically related to nitroglycerin, has been used for many years in the treatment and symptomatic relief of angina. It is also effective in the emergency management of cyanide poisoning. It is supplied in a glass inhalant that can be broken and inhaled immediately. Amyl nitrite causes the oxidation of hemoglobin to a compound called methemoglobin. Methemoglobin reacts with the toxic cyanide ion to form cyanomethemoglobin, which can be enzymatically degraded.

Indication

- Cyanide poisoning

Contraindications

There are no contraindications to the use of amyl nitrite in the management of cyanide poisoning.

Precautions

Headache and hypotension have been known to occur following the inhalation of amyl nitrite. Amyl nitrite is frequently abused and should be kept in a secure place with the narcotics.

Dosage

One to two inhalants of amyl nitrite should be crushed and inhaled. This should be maintained until the patient has reached an emergency department. Therapeutic effects diminish after approximately 20 minutes.

Route

Amyl nitrite should be administered by inhalation only.

How Supplied

Amyl nitrite is supplied in inhalants containing 0.3 milliliters.

OVERDOSE

Overdose with both prescribed and nonprescribed medications is common. Prehospital management of the overdose patient is aimed primarily at supportive care. In some cases, however, the administration of antidotes may be indicated.

The principal problem with medication overdose is depression of the central nervous system. Diminished level of consciousness and respiratory depression are commonly seen. Prehospital care should include immediate management of the airway, supplemental administration of oxygen, and placement of an intravenous line. If the suspected drug is a narcotic or narcotic-like agent, **naloxone** may be effective in reversing the respiratory depression. If the agent was atropine or one of the drugs with anticholinergic properties, like the tricyclic antidepressants, then **physostigmine** may be effective.

Naloxone (Narcan®)

Description

Naloxone is an effective narcotic antagonist and has proved effective in the management and reversal of overdoses caused by narcotics or synthetic narcotic agents. Recent studies have shown that naloxone may also be effective in reversal of coma associated with alcohol ingestion.

Indications

- For the complete or partial reversal of depression caused by narcotics including the following agents:

morphine	Demerol®
heroin	paregoric
Dilaudid®	codeine
Percodan®	Fentanyl®
methadone	

- For the complete or partial reversal of depression caused by synthetic narcotic analgesic agents including the following drugs:

Nubain®	Talwin®
Stadol®	Darvon®

- Alcoholic coma
- Treatment of coma of unknown origin

Contraindications

Naloxone should not be administered to a patient with a history of hypersensitivity to the drug.

Precautions

Naloxone should be administered cautiously to patients who are known or suspected to be physically dependent on narcotics. Abrupt and complete reversal by naloxone can cause withdrawal-type effects. This includes newborn infants of mothers with known or suspected narcotic dependence.

Dosage

The standard dosage for suspected or confirmed narcotic or synthetic narcotic overdoses is 1 to 2 milligrams IV. If unsuccessful, then a second dose may be administered 5 minutes later. Failure to obtain reversal after 2 to 3 doses indicates another disease process or overdosage on nonopioid drugs.

Larger than average doses (2 to 5 milligrams) have been used in the management of Darvon overdoses and alcoholic coma.

An intravenous infusion can be prepared by placing 2 milligrams of naloxone in 500 milliliters of D_5W. This gives a concentration of 4 micrograms per milliliter. One hundred milliliters per hour should be infused, thus delivering 0.4 milligrams per hour.

Route

In the emergency setting, naloxone should be administered intravenously only. When an IV line cannot be established, intramuscular or subcutaneous administration can be performed.

How Supplied

Naloxone is supplied in ampules and prefilled syringes containing 2 milligrams in 2 milliliters of solvent. In addition, vials containing 10 milliliters of the 1 milligram per milliliter concentration are also available.

Physostigmine (Antilirium®)

Description

Physostigmine is a potentially effective antidote for the management of poisonings resulting from atropine-type drugs and overdoses of tricyclic-type antidepressants. These drugs cause an increase in cholinesterase activity, thus inhibiting the action of acetylcholine in both parasympathetic and voluntary nerves. Physostigmine inhibits the destructive action of cholinesterase, thus exaggerating the effect of acetylcholine.

Atropine-type poisonings can result from an overdose of atropine or scopalamine. Several plants contain atropine-type chemicals. Ingestion of parts of these plants can cause anticholinergic poisoning.

Tricyclic poisoning occurs only following an overdose of the drugs within the tricyclic class. Tricyclic drugs are frequently prescribed for the management of depression. Overdoses of tricyclics are particularly dangerous because of serious effects they have on the heart. Cardiac arrhythmias, especially those indicative of conduction system disturbances, are common. Toxic doses of tricyclics result in cholinesterase inhibition. The administration of physostigmine is often effective in reversing the ill effects.

The administration of physostigmine to tricyclic overdose is controversial. Most authorities agree that alkalinization is the primary treatment. Local protocols should be followed regarding physostigmine usage.

Indications

- To reverse the toxic effects of the tricyclic class of antidepressants including the following:

Tofranil®	Adapin®
Norpramin®	Sinequan®
Elavil®	

- To reverse the toxic effects of atropine and atropine-like drugs including the following plants with belladonna agents present:

Pyrocantha	Lantana
Jimsonweed	Angel's Trumpet

Contraindications

Physostigmine should not be administered in the presence of asthma, gangrene, diabetes, or cardiovascular disease.

Precautions

If excessive parasympathetic actions are seen, such as increased salivation, or if emesis or bradycardia occurs, then the dosage of the drug should be reduced. IV administration should be at a slow and controlled rate. No more than 1 milligram per minute should be administered. Atropine sulfate should be on hand for use as an antagonist.

Dosage

The usual adult dosage is 0.5 to 2 milligrams slow IV bolus. It may be necessary to repeat the dose 5 minutes later if life-threatening signs reoccur.

Routes

Physostigmine should be given via slow IV bolus. When an IV line cannot be started, then intramuscular injection can be used.

How Supplied

Antilirium is supplied in 2-milliliter ampules containing 2 milligrams (1 milligram per milliliter).

SUMMARY

Treatment of toxicological emergencies is usually only supportive in the prehospital phase of emergency medical care. Several agents are effective in alleviation of the life-threatening effects of anaphylaxis, however. The primary drug in managing anaphylaxis is epinephrine. Benadryl and the common steroid preparations, Solu-Medrol and Solu-Cortef, may also be effective, however. Poisoning and overdoses should be treated symptomatically. Essential care includes airway maintenance, administration of supplemental oxygen, and establishment of an IV infusion. In addition, it is often necessary to reduce or prohibit the adsorbtion of the drug into the body. Syrup of ipecac and activated charcoal are often effective in accomplishing this. In addition, several antidotes are available to reverse the systemic effects of a great many agents.

12

DRUGS USED IN MANAGEMENT OF BEHAVIORAL EMERGENCIES

INTRODUCTION

Behavioral emergencies rarely require pharmacological intervention during the prehospital phase of emergency medical care. There are situations, however, in which emergency personnel may be called on to administer a sedative or similar agent. Among these are acute anxiety reactions and paranoid psychoses. Occasionally, it may be necessary to administer a sedative to friends or family of a patient who has been severely injured or who has recently died.

Common agents used in the acute treatment of behavioral emergencies include haloperidol (Haldol®), chlorpromazine (Thorazine®), and hydroxyzine (Vistaril®).

Haloperidol (Haldol®)

Description

Haloperidol is a frequently used major tranquilizer. It has proved effective in the management of acute psychotic episodes. It has pharmacological properties similar to those of the phenothiazine class of drugs (for example, Thorazine). Haloperidol is believed to block dopamine receptors in the brain associated with mood and behavior.

Indication

- Acute psychotic episodes

Contraindications

Haloperidol should not be administered in cases in which other drugs, especially sedatives, may be present. Haloperidol should not be used in the management of dysphoria caused by Talwin® as it may promote sedation and anesthesia.

Precautions

Haloperidol may impair mental and physical abilities. Occasionally, orthostatic hypotension may be seen in conjunction with haloperidol use. Caution should be used when administering haloperidol to patients on anticoagulants.

Extrapyramidal, or Parkinson-like, reactions have been known to occur following the administration of haloperidol, especially in children. Diphenhydramine should be readily available.

Dosage

Doses of 2 to 5 milligrams intramuscularly are fairly standard in the management of an acute psychotic episode with severe symptoms.

Route

Haloperidol should be given intramuscularly only.

How Supplied

Haloperidol is supplied in 1-milliliter ampules containing 5 milligrams of the drug.

Chlorpromazine (Thorazine®)

Description

Chlorpromazine is a major tranquilizer used in the management of severe psychotic episodes. It is a member of the phenothiazine class of drugs. Phenothiazine drugs are thought to block dopamine receptors in the brain associated with behavior and mood. Chlorpromazine is also effective in the management of mild alcohol withdrawal and intractible hiccoughs. It is also effective in reducing nausea and vomiting, although better agents are available.

Indications

- Acute psychotic episodes
- Mild alcohol withdrawal
- Intractible hiccoughs
- Nausea and vomiting

Contraindications

Chlorpromazine should not be administered to patients in comatose states or who have recently taken a large amount of sedatives. Chlorpromazine should not be administered to patients who may have recently taken hallucinogens as it tends to promote seizures.

Precautions

Chlorpromazine may impair mental and physical abilities. Occasionally, orthostatic hypotension may be seen in conjunction with chlorpromazine use.

Extrapyramidal, or Parkinson-like, reactions have been known to occur following the administration of chlorpromazine, especially in children. Diphenhydramine should be readily available.

Dosage

The standard dose of chlorpromazine in the management of an acute psychotic episode is 25 milligrams intramuscularly.

Route

Chlorpromazine should only be administered intramuscularly.

How Supplied

Chlorpromazine is supplied in 1- and 2-milliliter ampules containing 25 milligrams per milliliter.

Hydroxyzine (Vistaril®)

Description

Hydroxyzine is a versatile drug used frequently in emergency medicine. Chemically unrelated to the phenothiazines, hydroxyzine, because of its antihistamine properties, has been shown to exert a calming effect during acute psychotic states. It is an effective antiemetic and a muscle relaxant. When administered concurrently with many analgesics, it tends to potentiate their effects.

Indications

- To potentiate the effects of narcotics and synthetic narcotics
- Nausea and vomiting
- Anxiety reactions

Contraindications

Hydroxyzine should not be administered to any patient with a history of hypersensitivity to the drug.

Precautions

Hydroxyzine is given by intramuscular injection only. When administered concurrently with analgesics, the potentiating effects of hydroxyzine should be kept in mind and the total analgesic dose should be adjusted accordingly.

Dosage

The standard dosage of hydroxyzine in the management of an acute anxiety reaction is 50 to 100 milligrams intramuscularly.
    The standard antiemetic dose is 25 to 50 milligrams.

Route

Hydroxyzine should be administered by intramuscular injection. Localized burning is a common complaint following an injection of hydroxyzine.

How Supplied

Hydroxyzine is supplied in single-dose vials containing 25 or 50 milligrams in 1 milliliter. Because the vials resemble each other, it is important to recheck the label to assure the correct dose is delivered to the patient.

SUMMARY

It is important to consider and rule out physical causes for bizarre behavior before determining that a patient's disorder is of a psychiatric origin. Disorders such as diabetes, head injury, and alcohol intoxication can cause such bizarre behavior. The psychotic patient is best handled in an emergency department by personnel skilled in psychiatric intervention. Sometimes psychotic reactions may require pharmacological intervention before transport is possible, however.

13

OTHER EMERGENCY DRUGS

OTHER EMERGENCY DRUGS

The drugs presented in this chapter do not readily fit into the major categories into which this text is divided. They are included here to assure a complete compendium of prehospital emergency drugs.

Phenergan® is an antiemetic that is used in many emergency situations. It also is frequently used as an adjunctive agent to potentiate the actions of several analgesics.

Anectine®, an extremely potent and dangerous skeletal muscle relaxant, is occasionally used in some of the more progressive EMS systems to obtain total paralysis before endotracheal intubation.

Promethazine (Phenergan®)

Description

Promethazine is a phenothiazine with more antihistamine effects than chlorpromazine. It also possesses considerable anticholinergic activity. It is an effective and commonly used antiemetic. It, unlike hydroxyzine, can be given intravenously. It is often administered with analgesics, particularly narcotics, to potentiate their effect.

Indications

- Nausea and vomiting
- Motion sickness
- To potentiate the effects of analgesics

Contraindications

Promethazine is contraindicated in comatose states and in patients who have received a large amount of depressants. Also, it should not be administered to any patient with a history of hypersensitivity to the drug.

Precautions

Promethazine may impair mental and physical ability. Care must be taken to avoid accidental intra-arterial injection. It should never be administered subcutaneously.

Dosage

The standard dosage of promethazine in the management of nausea and vomiting is 12.5 to 25 milligrams either intravenously or intramuscularly.
    The standard dosage in adjunctive use with analgesics is 25 milligrams.

Routes

Promethazine should be given by IV or deep intramuscular injection only. Care must be taken to avoid accidental intra-arterial injection.

How Supplied

Promethazine is supplied in ampules and Tubex containing 25 milligrams of the drug in 1 milliliter of solvent.

Succinylcholine (Anectine®)

Description

Succinylcholine is a short-acting, depolarizing, skeletal muscle relaxant. Like acetylcholine, it combines with cholinergic receptors in the motor nerves to cause depolarization. Neuromuscular transmission is thus inhibited and remains so for 8 to 10 minutes.
    Following IV injection, complete paralysis is obtained within 1 minute and persists for approximately 2 minutes. Effects then start to fade, and a return to normal is seen within 6 minutes.

Muscle relaxation begins in the eyelids and jaw. It then progresses to the limbs, the abdomen, and finally the diaphragm and intercostals. It has no effect on the consciousness whatsoever.

Indication

- To achieve temporary paralysis where endotracheal intubation is indicated and where muscle tone or seizure activity prevents it

Contraindications

Succinylcholine is indicated in patients with a history of hypersensitivity to the drug.

Precautions

Succinylcholine should not be administered unless personnel skilled in endotracheal intubation are present and ready to perform the procedure. Oxygen therapy equipment should be readily available as should all emergency resuscitative drugs and equipment.

Dosage

The dosage for succinylcholine is 1 milligram per kilogram intravenously.

Route

The preferred route for succinylcholine administration is intravenously. It can be administered intramuscularly if required, however.

How Supplied

Succinylcholine is supplied in vials containing 10 milliliters of a 20 milligrams per milliliter concentration (200 total milligrams).

REFERENCES

AMERICAN HEART ASSOCIATION, *Textbook of Advanced Cardiac Life Support*, 2nd ed. Dallas, TX: American Heart Association, 1987.

AMERICAN HEART ASSOCIATION AND AMERICAN ACADEMY OF PEDIATRICS, *Textbook of Neonatal Resuscitation*. Dallas, TX: American Heart Association, 1987.

AMERICAN HEART ASSOCIATION AND AMERICAN ACADEMY OF PEDIATRICS, *Textbook of Pediatric Advanced Life Support*. Dallas, TX: American Heart Association, 1988.

BAYER, MARK J., RUMACK, BARRY H., AND WANKE, LEE A., *Toxicological Emergencies*, Bowie, MD: Brady Communications, 1984.

BLEDSOE, BRYAN E., PORTER, ROBERT S., AND SHADE, BRUCE, *Paramedic Emergency Care*. Englewood Cliffs, NJ: Prentice Hall, 1991.

BRAUNWALD, EUGENE, *Heart Disease: A Textbook of Cardiovascular Medicine*, 2nd ed. Philadelphia, PA: W. B. Saunders, 1984.

GOODMAN, L. S., AND GILMAN, A., *The Pharmacological Basis of Therapeutics*, 7th ed. New York: MacMillan, 1985.

HAMBURGER, STEPHEN, RUSH, DAVID R., AND BOSKER, GIDEON, *Endocrine and Metabolic Emergencies*, Bowie, MD: Brady Communications, 1984.

MEDICAL ECONOMICS COMPANY. *Physician's Desk Reference*, 45th ed. Oradell, NJ: Medical Economics Company, 1991.

SHADE, BRUCE, ET AL, *Advanced Cardiac Life Support: Certification, Preparation, and Review*. Englewood Cliffs, NJ: Brady Communications, 1988.

TINTINALLI, JUDITH E., KROME, RONALD L., AND RUIZ, ERNEST, *Emergency Medicine: A Comprehensive Study Guide*, 2nd ed. New York: McGraw-Hill, 1988.

UNITED STATES DEPARTMENT OF TRANSPORTATION, NATIONAL HIGHWAY TRAFFIC SAFETY ADMINISTRATION, *Emergency Medical Technician–Paramedic: National Standard Curriculum*. Washington, DC: U.S. Government Printing Office, 1985.

GLOSSARY

absorb—to take into the body.

acidosis—state in which the pH is lower than normal because of an increased hydrogen ion concentration.

acute myocardial infarction—death and subsequent necrosis of the heart muscle caused by inadequate blood supply.

addiction—physical or psychological dependence on a substance.

adrenergic—see *sympathomimetic*.

afterload—pressure or resistance against which the heart must pump.

agonist—drug or other substance that causes a physiological response.

air embolism—presence of an air bubble in the circulatory system.

albumin—protein found in all animal tissues that constitutes one of the major proteins in human blood.

alkalosis—state in which the pH is higher than normal because of a decreased hydrogen ion concentration.

allergic reaction—hypersensitivity to a given antigen; a reaction more pronounced than would occur in the general population.

amphetamine—substance that acts on the central nervous system as a stimulant.

anaphylaxis—acute, generalized, and violent antigen-antibody reaction that may be rapidly fatal.

antagonism—opposition of effect between two or more medications.

antagonist—drug or other substance that blocks a physiological response or that blocks the action of another drug or substance.

antiadrenergic—see *sympatholytic.*

antibiotics—medications effective in inhibiting the growth or killing of bacteria. They have no impact on viruses.

anticholinergic—see *parasympatholytic.*

antidote—substance that neutralizes a poison or the effects of a poison.

antigen—any substance capable of inducing an immune response.

apothecary's system—an antiquated system of weights and measures used widely in early medicine.

arrhythmia—absence of cardiac electrical activity, often used interchangeably with dysrhythmia.

autonomic nervous system—part of the nervous system controlling involuntary bodily functions; separated into the sympathetic and the parasympathetic divisions.

barbiturates—organic compounds derived from barbituric acid that depress the central nervous system, respirations, and heart rate, and decrease blood pressure.

benzodiazepines—general term to describe a group of tranquilizing drugs with similar chemical structures.

biotransformation—process of changing a drug into a different form, either active or inactive, by the body.

blood brain barrier—protective mechanism that selectively allows the entry of only a few compounds into brain.

bolus—single, oftentimes large, dose of a medication.

bradycardia—heart rate less than 60 beats per minute.

buffer—substance that neutralizes or weakens a strong acid or base.

cardiac contractile force—force generated by the heart during each contraction.

cardiac output—amount of blood pumped by the heart in 1 minute.

cardiogenic shock—inability of the heart to meet the metabolic needs of the body, resulting in inadequate tissue perfusion.

cardioversion—passage of a current through the heart during a specific part of the cardiac cycle to terminate certain dysrhythmias.

catecholamines—class of hormones that act on the autonomic nervous system including epinephrine, norepinephrine, and similar compounds.

cholinergic—see *parasympathomimetic*.

chronotrope—drug or other substance that affects the heart rate.

chronotropy—pertaining to heart rate.

colloid osmotic pressure—pressure generated by the presence of colloids in the vascular system or in interstitial spaces.

contraindications—medical or physiological conditions present in a patient that would make it harmful to administer a medication of otherwise known therapeutic value.

COPD—Chronic obstructive pulmonary disease characterized by a decreased ability of the lungs to perform the function of ventilation.

croup—laryngotracheobronchitis, a common viral infection of young children resulting in edema of the subglottic tissues; characterized by barking cough and inspiratory stridor.

defibrillation—the passage of a DC electrical current through a fibrillating heart to depolarize a "critical mass" of myocardial cells allowing them to depolarize uniformly, resulting in an organized rhythm.

dehydration—abnormal decrease in total body water.

delirium tremens (DTs)—disorder found in habitual and excessive users of alcoholic beverages after cessation of drinking for 48 to 72 hours; patients experience visual, tactile, and auditory hallucinations.

depressant—medication that decreases or lessens a body function.

diffusion—movement of solutes (substances dissolved in a solution) from an area of greater concentration to an area of lesser concentration.

drug—chemical agent used in diagnosis, treatment, and prevention of disease.

dysrhythmia—any deviation from the normal electrical rhythm of the heart.

electrolytes—chemical substances that dissociate into charged particles when placed in water.

endocrine gland—gland that secretes hormones directly into the blood.

epiglottitis—bacterial infection of the epiglottis, usually occurring in children older than age 4; a serious medical emergency.

FiO₂—concentration of oxygen in inspired air.

habituation—physical or psychological dependence on a drug.

half-life—time required for level of a drug in the blood to be reduced by 50 percent of its beginning level.

hematocrit—percentage of the blood consisting of the red blood cells, or erythrocytes (usually 35 to 45 percent).

histamine—chemical released by mast cells and basophils on stimulation; one of the most powerful vasodilators known and a major mediator of anaphylaxis.

homeostasis—body's natural tendency to keep the internal environment constant.

hormone—chemical substance released by a gland that controls or affects other glands or body systems.

hypersensitivity—reaction that is more profound than seen in the normal population.

hypertension—common disorder characterized by elevation of the blood pressure persistently exceeding 140/90 millimeters of mercury.

hypertensive emergency—acute elevation of blood pressure that requires the blood pressure be lowered within 1 hour, characterized by end-organ changes such as hypertensive encephalopathy, renal failure, or blindness.

hypertensive encephalopathy—cerebral disorder of hypertension indicated by severe headache, nausea, vomiting, and altered mental status; neurological symptoms may include blindness, muscle twitches, inability to speak, weakness, and paralysis.

hypertensive urgency—an acute elevation of blood pressure that requires the blood pressure to be lowered in 24 hours, usually unaccompanied by end-organ changes.

hypertonic—state in which a solution has a higher solute concentration on one side of a semipermeable membrane compared with the other side.

hypoglycemia—complication of diabetes characterized by low levels of blood glucose; often occurs from too high a dose of insulin or from inadequate food intake following a normal insulin dose; sometimes called insulin shock, hypoglycemia is a true medical emergency.

hypotonic—state in which a solution has a lower solute concentration on one side of a semipermeable membrane compared with the other side.

hypoxemia—reduction in the oxygen content in the arterial blood or in the PaO_2.

hypoxia—state in which insufficient oxygen is available to meet the oxygen requirements of the cells.

idiosyncrasy—reaction to a drug that is unusually different from that seen in the rest of the population.

indication—medical condition(s) in which a drug has proved to be of therapeutic value.

ingestion—entrance of a substance into the body through the gastrointestinal tract.

inhalation—entrance of a substance into the body through the respiratory tract.

injection—entrance of a substance into the body through a break in the skin.

inotrope—drug or other substance that affects the contractile force of the heart.

inotropy—pertaining to cardiac contractile force.

intractable—resistant to cure, relief, or control.

intraosseous injection—to administer into the bone marrow, an alternative to venous access in children under the age of 2 years.

isotonic—state in which solutions on opposite sides of a semipermeable membrane are in equal concentration.

ketoacidosis—complication of diabetes owing to decreased insulin secretion or intake, which is characterized by high levels of glucose in the blood, metabolic acidosis, and, in advanced stages, coma; ketoacidosis is often called diabetic coma.

Korsakoff's syndrome—psychosis characterized by disorientation, muttering delirium, insomnia, delusions, and hallucinations; symptoms include painful extremities, bilateral wrist drop (rarely), bilateral foot drop (frequently), and pain or pressure over the long nerves.

logarithm—mathematical concept that eases calculation of large numbers; the log of a number is the exponent of the power to which a given base must be raised to equal that number—for example, the log of 100 is 2 ($100 = 10^2$), and the log of 1000 is 3 ($1000 = 10^3$).

metric system—system of weights and measures widely used in science and medicine, and based on a base unit of 10.

milliequivalent—number of grams of a solute contained in 1 milliliter of a normal solution.

neurotransmitter—substance that is released from the axon terminal of a presynaptic neuron on excitation that travels across the synaptic cleft to either excite or inhibit the target cell; examples include acetylcholine, norepinephrine, and dopamine.

osmosis—movement of a solvent (water) across a semipermeable membrane from an area of lesser (solute) concentration to an area of greater (solute) concentration; osmosis is a form of diffusion.

overdose—dose of a drug in excess of that usually prescribed, which can potentially adversely affect the patient's health.

overhydration—excess of total body water.

parasympathetic nervous system—division of the autonomic nervous system that is responsible for controlling vegetative functions.

parasympatholytic—drug or other substance that blocks or inhibits the actions of the parasympathetic nervous system (also called anticholinergic).

parasympathomimetic—drug or other substance that causes effects like those of the parasympathetic nervous system (also called cholinergic).

parenteral drugs—drugs administered into the body without going through the digestive tract are referred to as parenteral drugs.

peripheral vascular resistance—resistance to blood flow owing to the peripheral blood vessels; this pressure must be overcome for the heart to pump blood effectively.

pH—scientific method of expressing the acidity or alkalinity of a solution, which is the logarithm of the hydrogen ion concentration divided by 1; the higher the pH the more alkaline the solution, and the lower the pH the more acidic the solution.

pharmacodynamics—study of a drug's action on the body.

pharmacokinetics—study of how drugs enter the body, reach their site of action, and are eventually eliminated.

pharmacology—study of drugs and how they affect the body.

physiology—study of body function.

plasma—fluid portion of the blood consisting of serum and protein substances in solution.

Poiseuille's law—law of physiology that states that blood flow through a vessel is directly proportional to the diameter of the vessel to the fourth power.

poison control center—information center staffed by trained personnel that provides up-to-date toxicological information.

poisoning—taking any substance into the body that interferes with normal physiological functions.

postpartum—period after delivery of the fetus.

preload—pressure within the ventricles at the end of diastole, commonly called the end-diastolic volume.

psychosis—any major mental disorder of organic or emotional origin, which is usually evidenced by derangement of the personality or loss of contact with reality.

refractory—disorder or condition that resists treatment.

seizure—disorder of the nervous system owing to a sudden, excessive, disorderly discharge of brain neurons.

semipermeable membrane—specialized biological membrane, such as that which encloses the body's cells, which allows the passage of certain substances and restricts the passage of others.

shock—state of inadequate tissue perfusion.

side effects—unavoidable, undesirable effects frequently seen even in therapeutic drug dosages.

status epilepticus—act of having two or more seizures in succession without intervening periods of consciousness.

stimulant—drug that enhances a bodily function.

surface absorption—entrance of a substance into the body directly through the skin.

sympathetic nervous system—division of the autonomic nervous system that prepares the body for stressful situations.

sympatholytic—drug or other substance that blocks the actions of the sympathetic nervous system (also called antiadrenergic).

sympathomimetic—drug or other substance that causes effects like those of the sympathetic nervous system (also called adrenergic).

syncope—transient loss of consciousness caused by inadequate blood flow to the brain.

synergism—combined action of two drugs that is much stronger than the effects of either drug administered separately.

tachycardia—heart rate greater than 100 beats per minute.

therapeutic action—desired, intended action of a drug given in the appropriate medical condition.

therapeutic index—index of a drug's safety profile, which is determined by calculating the difference between the drug's therapeutic threshold and toxic level. It is typically determined in the laboratory.

therapeutic threshold—minimum amount of drug needed in the bloodstream to cause the desired therapeutic effect.

titration—estimation of the appropriate dosage by slowly changing the rate of administration.

tonicity—number of particles present per unit volume.

universal precautions—set of procedures and precautions published by the Centers for Disease Control to assist health care personnel in protecting themselves from infectious disease.

Valsalva's maneuver—forced exhalation against a closed glottis that increases the intra-abdominal and intrathoracic pressure, causing slowing of the pulse.

Wernicke's syndrome—condition characterized by loss of memory and disorientation, associated with chronic alcohol intake and a diet deficient in thiamine.

Wolff-Parkinson-White syndrome—disorder of the heart characterized by early contraction of part of the heart muscle.

APPENDIX A

QUICK DRUG REFERENCE

INTRODUCTION

This section provides a quick reference to more than seventy of the most commonly used emergency medications. The dosages and indications have been taken from the most recent Advanced Cardiac Life Support (ACLS) standards of the American Heart Association. Drugs not covered in ACLS are taken from the American Medical Association's *Drug Evaluation*. It is important to remember that specific drugs, dosages, indications, and routes may vary in your particular area. It is essential to be familiar with these variations and follow the guidelines established by the medical director of the system in which you work.

Activated Charcoal	
Class:	Adsorbent
Action:	Adsorbs toxins by chemical binding and prevents gastrointestinal adsorption
Indications:	Poisoning following emesis or when emesis is contraindicated
Contraindications:	None in severe poisoning

Precautions:	Should only be administered following emesis in cases in which it is so indicated
	Use with caution in patients with altered mental status
	May adsorb ipecac before emesis; if ipecac is administered, wait at least 10 minutes to administer activated charcoal
Side Effects:	Nausea, vomiting, and constipation
Dosage:	0.5–1 g/kg mixed with a glass of water to form a slurry
Route:	Oral
Pediatric Dosage:	0.5–1 g/kg mixed with a glass of water to form a slurry

---

Adenosine (Adenocard®)

Class:	Antiarrhythmic
Action:	Slows AV conduction
Indications:	Symptomatic PSVT
Contraindications:	Second- or third-degree heart block
	Sick-sinus syndrome
	Known hypersensitivity to the drug
Precautions:	Arrhythmias, including blocks, are common at the time of cardioversion
	Use with caution in patients with asthma
Side Effects:	Facial flushing, headache, shortness of breath, dizziness, and nausea
Dosage:	6 mg given as a rapid IV bolus over a 1–2-second period; if, after 1–2 minutes, cardioversion does not occur, administer a 12-mg dose over 1–2 seconds
Route:	IV; should be administered directly into a vein or into the medication administration port closest to the patient and followed by flushing of the line with IV fluid
Pediatric Dosage:	Safety in children has not been established

Albuterol (Proventil®) (Ventolin®)

Class:	Sympathomimetic (β_2 selective)
Action:	Bronchodilation
Indications:	Asthma Reversible bronchospasm associated with COPD
Contraindications:	Known hypersensitivity to the drug Symptomatic tachycardia
Precautions:	Blood pressure, pulse, and EKG should be monitored Use caution in patients with known heart disease
Side Effects:	Palpitations, anxiety, headache, dizziness, and sweating
Dosage:	*Metered-Dose Inhaler* 1–2 sprays (90-µg per spray) *Small-Volume Nebulizer* 0.5 ml (2.5 mg) in 2.5 ml normal saline over 5–15 minutes *Rotohaler* One 200-µg Rotocap should be placed in the inhaler and breathed by the patient
Route:	Inhalation
Pediatric Dosage:	0.15 mg (0.03 ml)/kg in 2.5 ml normal saline

Aminophylline

Class:	Xanthine bronchodilator
Actions:	Smooth muscle relaxant Causes bronchodilation Has mild diuretic properties Increases heart rate
Indications:	Bronchial asthma Reversible bronchospasm associated with chronic bronchitis and emphysema Congestive heart failure Pulmonary edema

Contraindications:	Patients with history of hypersensitivity to the drug Hypotension Patients with peptic ulcer disease
Precautions:	Monitor for arrhythmias Monitor blood pressure Do not administer to patients on chronic theophylline preparations until the theophylline blood level has been determined
Side Effects:	Convulsions, tremor, anxiety, and dizziness Vomiting Palpitations, PVCs, and tachycardia
Dosages:	*Method 1* 250–500 mg in 90 or 80 ml of D$_5$W, respectively, infused over 20–30 minutes (approximately 5–10 mg/kg/hr) *Method 2* 250–500 mg (5–7 mg/kg) in 20 ml of D$_5$W infused over 20–30 minutes
Route:	Slow IV infusion
Pediatric Dosage:	5–6 mg/kg loading dose to be infused over 20–30 minutes; maximum dose not to exceed 12 mg/kg per 24 hours

---

Amrinone (Inocor®)

Class:	Cardiac inotrope
Actions:	Increases cardiac contractility Vasodilator
Indications:	Short-term management of congestive heart failure not associated with myocardial infarction
Contraindications:	Patients with history of hypersensitivity to the drug Patients suffering congestive heart failure following myocardial infarction
Precautions:	May increase myocardial ischemia Blood pressure, pulse, and EKG should be constantly monitored

Amrinone should only be diluted with normal saline or 1/2 normal saline; no dextrose solutions should be used

Furosemide (Lasix®) should not be administered into an IV line delivering amrinone

Side Effects:	Reduction in platelets Nausea and vomiting Cardiac arrhythmias
Dosage:	0.75 mg/kg bolus given slowly over 2–3-minute interval followed by maintenance infusion of 2–20 µg/kg minute
Route:	IV bolus and infusion as described earlier
Pediatric Dosage:	Safety in children has not been established

---

Amyl Nitrite

Class:	Nitrate
Actions:	Causes coronary vasodilation Removes cyanide-ion via complex mechanism
Indications:	Cyanide poisoning (bitter almond smell to breath)
Contraindications:	None when used in the management of cyanide poisoning
Precautions:	Hypotension common Has tendency for abuse
Side Effects:	Headache Hypotension, reflex tachycardia Nausea
Dosage:	Inhalant should be broken and inhaled, repeated as needed until patient is delivered to emergency department; effects diminish after 20 minutes
Route:	Inhalation
Pediatric Dosage:	Inhalant should be broken and inhaled, repeated until patient is delivered to emergency department

Atropine

Class:	Parasympatholytic (anticholinergic)
Actions:	Blocks acetylcholine receptors Increases heart rate Decreases gastrointestinal secretions
Indications:	Bradycardia Hypotension secondary to bradycardia Third-degree heart block Asystole Organophosphate poisoning
Contraindications:	None when used in emergency situations
Precautions:	Dose of 2.0 mg should not be exceeded except in cases of organophosphate poisonings Tachycardia Hypertension
Side Effects:	Palpitations and tachycardia Headache, dizziness, and anxiety Dry mouth, pupillary dilation, and blurred vision Urinary retention (especially older males)
Dosage:	*Bradycardia* 0.5 mg every 5 minutes to maximum of 2.0 mg *Asystole* 1 mg *Organophosphate Poisoning* 2–5 mg
Route:	IV Endotracheal
Pediatric Dosage:	*Bradycardia* 0.01–0.03 mg/kg *Organophosphate Poisoning* 0.05 mg/kg

Bretylium (Bretylol®)

Class:	Antiarrhythmic

Action:	Increases ventricular fibrillation threshold Blocks the release of norepinephrine from peripheral sympathetic nerves
Indications:	Ventricular fibrillation refractory to lidocaine Ventricular tachycardia refractory to lidocaine PVCs refractory to first-line medications
Contraindications:	None when used in the management of life-threatening arrhythmias
Precautions:	Postural hypotension occurs in approximately 50 percent of patients receiving Bretylium Patient must be kept supine Decrease dosage in patients being treated with catecholamine sympathomimetics
Side Effects:	Hypotension, syncope, and bradycardia Increased frequency of arrhythmias Dizziness and vertigo
Dosage:	5 mg/kg May be repeated at dose of 10 mg/kg up to a total dose of 30 mg/kg
Route:	Rapid IV bolus
Pediatric Dosage:	Safety in children has not been established

---

Bumetanide (Bumex®)

Class:	Potent diuretic
Actions:	Inhibits reabsorption of sodium chloride Promotes prompt diuresis Slight vasodilation
Indications:	Congestive heart failure Pulmonary edema
Contraindications:	Dehydration Pregnancy
Precautions:	Should be protected from light Dehydration
Side Effects:	Few in emergency usage
Dosage:	0.5–1.0 mg

Routes:	IV
	Intramuscular
Pediatric Dosage:	Safety in children has not been established

---

Butorphanol (Stadol®)

Class:	Synthetic analgesic
Actions:	Central nervous system depressant
	Decreases sensitivity to pain
	2 mg Stadol® equivalent to 10 mg morphine
Indications:	Moderate to severe pain
Contraindications:	Patients with a history of hypersensitivity to the drug
	Head injury
	Use with caution in patients with impaired respiratory function
Precautions:	Respiratory depression (Narcan® should be available)
	Patients dependent on narcotics
Side Effects:	May experience symptoms of withdrawal
	Nausea
	Altered levels of consciousness
Dosage:	IV
	1 mg
	Intramuscular
	2 mg
Routes:	IV
	Intramuscular
Pediatric Dosage:	Rarely used

Calcium Chloride

Class:	Electrolyte
Actions:	Increases cardiac contractility
Indications:	Acute hyperkalemia (elevated potassium)
	Acute hypocalcemia (decreased calcium)

Calcium channel blocker (nifedipine, verapamil, etc.) overdose
Abdominal muscle spasm associated with spider bite and Portuguese man-o-war stings

Contraindications: Patients receiving digitalis

Precautions: IV line should be flushed between calcium chloride and sodium bicarbonate administration
Extravasation may cause tissue necrosis

Side Effects: Arrhythmias (bradycardia and asystole)
Hypotension

Dosage: 2–4 mg/kg of a 10% solution; may be repeated at 10-minute intervals

Route: IV

Pediatric Dosage: 5–7 mg/kg of a 10% solution

| Chlorpromazine (Thorazine®) |

Class: Major tranquilizer

Actions: Blocks dopamine receptors in brain associated with mood and behavior
Has antiemetic properties

Indications: Acute psychotic episodes
Mild alcohol withdrawal
Intractable hiccoughs
Nausea and vomiting

Contraindications: Comatose states
Should not be administered in the presence of sedatives
Should not be administered in the presence of hallucinogens or phencyclidine-like compounds

Precautions: Orthostatic hypotension
May cause extrapyramidal reactions (Parkinson-like), especially in children

Side Effects: Physical and mental impairment
Drowsiness

Dosage: 25–100 mg

Route: Intramuscular

Pediatric Dosage: 0.5 mg/kg

Dexamethasone (Decadron®, Hexadrol®)

Class: Steroid

Actions: Decreases cerebral edema
                        Anti-inflammatory
                        Suppresses immune response (especially in al-
                            lergic reactions)

Indications: Cerebral edema
                        Anaphylaxis (after epinephrine and diphenhydra-
                            mine)

Contraindications: None in the emergency setting

Precautions: Should be protected from heat
                        Onset of action may be 2–6 hours and thus should
                            not be considered to be of use in the critical
                            first hour following an anaphylactic reaction

Side Effects: Gastrointestinal bleeding
                        Prolonged wound healing

Dosage: 4–24 mg

Route: IV

Pediatric Dosage: 0.2–0.5 mg/kg

50% Dextrose

Class: Carbohydrate

Actions: Elevates blood glucose level rapidly

Indications: Hypoglycemia
                        Coma of unknown origin

Contraindications: None in the emergency setting

Precautions: A blood sample should be drawn before admin-
                            istering 50% dextrose

Side Effects: Local venous irritation

Dosage:	25 grams (50 ml)
Route:	IV
Pediatric Dosage:	0.5–1 g/kg slow IV; should be diluted 1:1 with sterile water to form a 25% solution

---

Diazepam (Valium®)

Class:	Tranquilizer
Actions:	Anticonvulsant
	Skeletal muscle relaxant
	Sedative
Indications:	Generalized seizures
	Status epilepticus
	Premedication before cardioversion
	Skeletal muscle relaxant
	Acute anxiety states
Contraindications:	Patients with a history of hypersensitivity to the drug
Precautions:	Can cause local venous irritation
	Has short duration of effect
	Do not mix with other drugs because of possible precipitation problems
Side Effects:	Drowsiness
	Hypotension
	Respiratory depression, apnea
Dosage:	*Status Epilepticus*
	5–10 mg IV
	Acute Anxiety
	2–5 mg intramuscular or IV
	Premedication before Cardioversion
	5–15 mg IV
Routes:	IV (care must be taken not to administer faster than 1 ml/min)
	Intramuscular
	Rectal
Pediatric Dosage:	*Status Epilepticus*
	0.5–2.0 mg

Diazoxide (Hyperstat®)

Class:	Antihypertensive
Actions:	Causes decrease in both systolic and diastolic pressures Direct peripheral arterial dilation
Indications:	Hypertensive emergency
Contraindications:	None in the emergency setting
Precautions:	Avoid overcorrection of blood pressure Blood pressure must be constantly monitored Patient should be supine
Side Effects:	Hypotension Syncope Local venous irritation
Dosage:	1–3 mg/kg boluses by rapid injection (less than 30 seconds) repeated at 5–15-minute intervals up to 150 mg in a single injection
Route:	IV only
Pediatric Dosage:	1–3 mg/kg

Digoxin (Lanoxin®)

Class:	Cardiac glycoside
Actions:	Increases cardiac contractile force Increases cardiac output Reduces edema associated with congestive heart failure Slows AV conduction
Indications:	Congestive heart failure Rapid atrial arrhythmias, especially atrial flutter and atrial fibrillation
Contraindications:	Any patient with signs or symptoms of digitalis toxicity Ventricular fibrillation
Precautions:	Monitor for signs of digitalis toxicity

Patients who have recently suffered a myocardial infarction have greater sensitivity to the effects of digitalis

Calcium should not be administered to patients receiving digitalis

Side Effects: Nausea
Vomiting
Arrhythmias
Yellow vision

Dosage: 0.25–0.50 mg

Route: IV

Pediatric Dosage: 25–40 µg/kg

| Diphenhydramine (Benadryl®) |

Class: Antihistamine

Actions: Blocks histamine receptors
Has some sedative effects

Indications: Anaphylaxis
Allergic reactions
Dystonic reactions due to phenothiazines

Contraindications: Asthma
Nursing mothers

Precautions: Hypotension

Side Effects: Sedation
Dries bronchial secretions
Blurred vision
Headache
Palpitations

Dosage: 25–50 mg

Routes: Slow IV push
Deep intramuscular

Pediatric Dosage: 2–5 mg/kg

Dobutamine (Dobutrex®)

Class:	Sympathomimetic
Actions:	Increases cardiac contractility Little chronotropic activity
Indications:	Short-term management of congestive heart failure
Contraindications:	Should only be used in patients with an adequate heart rate
Precautions:	Ventricular irritability Use with caution following myocardial infarction Can be deactivated by alkaline solutions
Side Effects:	Increased heart rate Palpitations
Dosage:	2.5–20 µg/kg/minute *Method* 250 mg should be placed in 500 ml of D_5W, which gives a concentration of 0.5 mg/ml
Route:	IV drip
Pediatric Dosage:	5–10 µg/kg/min

Dopamine (Intropin®)

Class:	Sympathomimetic
Actions:	Increases cardiac contractility Causes peripheral vasoconstriction
Indications:	Cardiogenic shock Hypovolemic shock (only after complete fluid resuscitation)
Contraindications:	Hypovolemic shock where complete fluid resuscitation has not occurred
Precautions:	Should not be administered in the presence of severe tachyarrhythmias Should not be administered in the presence of ventricular fibrillation Ventricular irritability

Side Effects:	Ventricular tachyarrhythmias
	Hypertension
Dosage:	2–10 μg/kg/minute; increase as needed
	Method
	800 mg should be placed in 500 ml of D_5W giving a concentration of 1600 μg/ml
Route:	IV drip only
Pediatric Dosage:	2–20 μg/kg/minute

Edrophonium (Tensilon®)

Class:	Anticholinesterase
Actions:	Inhibits action of enzyme cholinesterase, thus potentiating acetylcholine
	Increases parasympathetic tone
Indications:	PSVT refractory to vagal maneuvers; considered a second-line agent to verapamil or adenosine
Contraindications:	Patients with a history of hypersensitivity to the drug
Precautions:	Respirations must be constantly monitored
	Bradycardia
	Hypotension
	Avoid exposure to dextrose solutions
Side Effects:	Dizziness
	Syncope
Dosage:	5 mg
Route:	IV
Pediatric Dosage:	0.1–0.2 mg/kg

Epinephrine 1:1000

Class:	Sympathomimetic
Actions:	Bronchodilation
Indications:	Bronchial asthma
	Exacerbation of COPD
	Allergic reactions

Contraindications:	Patients with underlying cardiovascular disease
	Hypertension
	Pregnancy
	Patients with tachyarrhythmias
Precautions:	Should be protected from light
	Blood pressure, pulse, and EKG must be constantly monitored
Side Effects:	Palpitations and tachycardia
	Anxiousness
	Headache
	Tremor
Dosage:	0.3–0.5 mg
Route:	Subcutaneous
Pediatric Dosage:	0.01 mg/kg up to 0.3 mg

Epinephrine 1:10,000

Class:	Sympathomimetic
Actions:	Increases heart rate
	Increases cardiac contractility
	Causes bronchodilation
Indications:	Cardiac arrest
	Anaphylactic shock
Contraindications:	None when used in the situations listed earlier
Precautions:	Should be protected from light
	Can be deactivated by alkaline solutions
Side Effects:	Tachyarrhythmias
	Palpitations
Dosage:	*Cardiac Arrest*
	0.5–1.0 mg repeated every 5 minutes
	Severe Anaphylaxis
	0.3–0.5 mg (3–5 ml)
Routes:	IV
	Endotracheal
Pediatric Dosage:	0.01 mg/kg repeated very 5 minutes

Epinephrine Suspension (Sus-Phrine®)

Class:	Sympathomimetic
Actions:	Bronchodilation Increases heart rate Increases cardiac contractility
Indications:	Bronchial asthma Allergic reaction
Contraindications:	Patients with underlying cardiovascular disease Pregnancy Patients with tachyarrhythmias
Precautions:	Should be protected from light Blood pressure, pulse, and EKG must be constantly monitored
Side Effects:	Palpitations, tachycardia Anxiousness Headache Tremor
Dosage:	0.1–0.3 ml
Route:	Subcutaneous
Pediatric Dosage:	0.005 ml/kg

Class:	Beta Blocker (β_1 selective)
Action:	Decreases heart rate Decreases AV conduction
Indications:	Symptomatic supraventricular tachycardia (including atrial fibrillation and atrial flutter) as evidenced by chest pain, palpitations, or dizziness
Contraindications:	Sinus bradycardia Heart block greater than first degree Cardiogenic shock Overt congestive heart failure Patients with bronchospastic disease (asthma)

Precautions:	Hypotension is common, usually dose related
	Patients with CHF may have worsening of their symptoms
	May worsen bronchospastic disease
Side Effects:	Dizziness, diaphoresis, and hypotension
	Nausea
Dosage:	*Preparation*
	Place two 2.5-gram ampules in 500 ml D_5W yielding a concentration of 10 mg/ml
	Loading Dose
	500 µg/kg/min for 1 minute; then reduce to maintenance dose
	Maintenance Dose
	50 µg/kg/min; if ineffective after 4 minutes, repeat loading dose and increase maintenance dose to 100 µg/kg/min; may repeat as needed until a total maintenance dose of 200 µg/kg/minute has been achieved
Route:	IV infusion only
Pediatric Dosage:	Safety in children has not been established

Furosemide (Lasix®)

Class:	Potent diuretic
Actions:	Inhibits reabsorption of sodium chloride
	Promotes prompt diuresis
	Vasodilation
Indications:	Congestive heart failure
	Pulmonary edema
Contraindications:	Pregnancy
	Dehydration
Precautions:	Should be protected from light
	Dehydration
Side Effects:	Few in emergency usage
Dosage:	40–80 mg
Route:	IV
Pediatric Dosage:	1 mg/kg

Glucagon

Class:	Hormone (antihypoglycemic agent)
Actions:	Causes breakdown of glycogen to glucose
	Inhibits glycogen synthesis
	Elevates blood glucose level
	Increases cardiac contractile force
	Increases heart rate
Indications:	Hypoglycemia
Contraindications:	Hypersensitivity to the drug
Precautions:	Only effective if there are sufficient stores of glycogen within the liver
	Use with caution in patients with cardiovascular or renal disease
	Draw blood glucose before administration
Side Effects:	Few in emergency situations
Dosage:	0.5–1.0 mg (unit)
Routes:	IV
	Intramuscular
Pediatric Dosage:	0.03 mg/kg

Glucola

Class:	Carbohydrate
Actions:	Increases blood glucose level
Indications:	Conscious patients with suspected hypoglycemia
Contraindications:	Any patient who is not conscious enough to drink without assistance
Precautions:	Monitor airway
	Draw blood glucose before administration
Side Effects:	Nausea
	Vomiting
Dosage:	Sipped until patient feels improvement (50–200 ml)

Route:	Oral
Pediatric Dosage:	Sipped until patient feels improvement

Haloperidol (Haldol®)

Class:	Major tranquilizer
Actions:	Blocks dopamine receptors in brain responsible for mood and behavior Has antiemetic properties
Indications:	Acute psychotic episodes
Contraindications:	Should not be administered in the presence of other sedatives Should not be used in the management of dysphoria caused by Talwin
Precautions:	Orthostatic hypotension
Side Effects:	Physical and mental impairment Parkinson-like reactions have been known to occur, especially in children
Dosage:	2–5 mg
Route:	Intramuscular
Pediatric Dosage:	Rarely used

Hydralazine (Apresoline®)

Class:	Antihypertensive (potent vasodilator)
Actions:	Relaxes vascular smooth muscle Decreased arterial pressure (diastolic greater than systolic) Increases cardiac output
Indications:	Hypertensive emergency in which a prompt reduction in blood pressure is required Hypertension accompanying pregnancy
Contraindications:	Patients with a known history of coronary artery disease Rheumatic heart disease involving the mitral valve History of hypersensitivity to the drug

Precautions:	May induce angina May cause EKG changes and cardiac ischemia Blood pressure, pulse rate, and EKG should be constantly monitored
Side Effects:	Headache, nausea, vomiting, tachycardia, palpitations, and diarrhea
Dosage:	20–40 mg given by slow IV bolus May be repeated, if required
Route:	IV
Pediatric Dosage:	Safety in children has not been established

---

Hydrocortisone (Solu-Cortef®)

Class:	Steroid
Actions:	Anti-inflammatory Suppresses immune response (especially in allergic/anaphylactic reactions)
Indications:	Severe anaphylaxis
Contraindications:	None in the emergency setting
Precautions:	Must be reconstituted and used promptly Onset of action may be 2–6 hours and thus should not be expected to be of use in the critical first hour following an acute anaphylactic reaction
Side Effects:	GI bleeding Prolonged wound healing Suppression of natural steroids
Dosage:	100–250 mg
Routes:	IV Intramuscular
Pediatric Dosage:	30 μg/kg

Hydroxyzine (Vistaril®)

Class:	Antihistamine

Actions:	Antiemetic Antihistamine Antianxiety Potentiates analgesic effects of narcotics and re- lated agents
Indications:	To potentiate the effects of narcotics and synthetic narcotics Nausea and vomiting Anxiety reactions
Contraindications:	Patients with a history of hypersensitivity to the drug
Precautions:	Orthostatic hypotension Analgesic dosages should be reduced when used with hydroxyzine Urinary retention
Side Effects:	Drowsiness
Dosage:	50–100 mg
Route:	Deep intramuscular only
Pediatric Dosage:	1 mg/kg

Insulin

Class:	Hormone (hypoglycemic agent)
Actions:	Causes uptake of glucose by the cells Decreases blood glucose level Promotes glucose storage
Indications:	Diabetic ketoacidosis
Contraindications:	Avoid overcompensation of blood glucose level; if possible, administration should wait until the patient is in the emergency department
Precautions:	Administration of excessive dose may induce hypoglycemia Glucose should be available
Side Effects:	Few in emergency situations
Dosage:	10–25 units regular insulin IV followed by an infusion at 0.1 units/kg/hr

Routes:	IV Subcutaneous
Pediatric Dosage:	Dosage is based on blood glucose level

Ipecac

Class:	Emetic
Actions:	Irritates the enteric tract Acts on vomiting center in the brain
Indications:	Poisoning in conscious patient
Contraindications:	Vomiting should not be induced in any patient with impaired consciousness Poisonings involving strong acids, bases, or petroleum distillates Antiemetic poisonings, especially of the phenothiazine type
Precautions:	Monitor and assure a patent airway The risk of aspiration is increased when using ipecac
Side Effects:	Rare
Dosage:	30 ml (1 ounce) followed by 15 ml/kg of warm water
Route:	Oral
Pediatric Dosage:	*Less Than 1 Year of Age* 10 ml *1–12 Years of Age* 15 ml *Greater Than 12 Years of Age* 30 ml

---

Isoetharine (Bronkosol®)

Class:	Sympathomimetic (β_2 selective)
Actions:	Bronchodilation Increases heart rate

Indications:	Asthma Reversible bronchospasm associated with chronic bronchitis and emphysema
Contraindications:	Patients with history of hypersensitivity to the drug
Precautions:	Blood pressure, pulse, and EKG must be constantly monitored
Side Effects:	Palpitations, tachycardia Anxiety and tremors Headache
Dosage:	*Hand Nebulizer* Four inhalations *Small-Volume Nebulizer* 0.5 ml (1:3 with saline)
Route:	Inhalation only
Pediatric Dosage:	0.25–0.5 ml diluted with 4 ml normal saline

---

Isoproterenol (Isuprel®)

Class:	Sympathomimetic
Actions:	Increases heart rate Increases cardiac contractile force Causes bronchodilation
Indications:	Bradycardias refractory to atropine Bradycardias due to high-degree heart blocks
Contraindications:	Should not be used to increase blood pressure in cardiogenic shock
Precautions:	Can cause ventricular irritability Can be deactivated by alkaline solutions Should be used with caution for recent myocardial infarction External pacing, if available, should be used instead of isoproterenol
Side Effects:	Tachyarrhythmias and tremor Palpitations and headache

Dosage:	1 mg should be placed in 500 ml of D_5W. This should then be slowly infused at 2–10 µg/min and titrated until the desired rate is obtained or until PVCs occur.
Route:	IV drip only
Pediatric Dosage:	0.1 µg/kg/minute

Labetalol (Trandate®) (Normodyne®)

Class:	Sympathetic blocker
Actions:	Selectively blocks α_1 receptors and nonselectively blocks β receptors
Indications:	Hypertensive crisis
Contraindications:	Bronchial asthma Congestive heart failure Heart block Bradycardia Cardiogenic shock
Precautions:	Blood pressure, pulse, and EKG must be constantly monitored Atropine and isoproterenol should be available
Side Effects:	Bradycardia Heart block Congestive heart failure Bronchospasm Postural hypotension
Dosage:	20 mg by slow IV infusion over 2 minutes; doses of 40 mg can be repeated in 10 minutes until desired supine blood pressure is obtained or until 300 mg of the drug has been given 200 mg placed in 500 ml D_5W to deliver 2 mg/minute
Route:	IV infusion or slow IV bolus as described earlier
Pediatric Dosage:	Safety in children has not been established

Lidocaine (Xylocaine®)

Class: Antiarrhythmic

Actions: Suppresses ventricular ectopic activity
Increases ventricular fibrillation threshold
Reduces velocity of electrical impulse through conductive system

Indications: Malignant PVCs
Ventricular tachycardia
Ventricular fibrillation
Prophylaxis of arrhythmias associated with acute myocardial infarction

Contraindications: High-degree heart blocks
PVCs in conjunction with bradycardia

Precautions: Dosage should not exceed 300 mg/hr
Monitor for central nervous system toxicity
Dosage should be reduced by 50% in patients older than 70 years of age or who have liver disease
Use bolus therapy only in cardiac arrest

Side Effects: Anxiety, drowsiness, dizziness, and confusion
Nausea and vomiting
Convulsions
Widening of QRS

Dosage: *Bolus*
Initial bolus of 1 mg/kg; additional boluses of 0.5 mg/kg can be repeated at 8–10-minute intervals until the arrhythmia has been suppressed or until 3 mg/kg of the drug has been administered; reduce dosage by 50% in patients older than 70 years of age
Drip
After the arrhythmia has been suppressed a 2–4-mg/minute infusion may be started to maintain adequate blood levels

Routes: IV bolus
IV infusion

Pediatric Dosage: 1 mg/kg

Magnesium Sulfate

Class:	Anticonvulsant
Actions:	Central nervous system depressant Anticonvulsant
Indications:	Eclampsia (toxemia of pregnancy)
Contraindications:	Any patient with heart block or recent myocardial infarction
Precautions:	Caution should be used in patients receiving digitalis Hypotension Calcium chloride should be readily available as an antidote if respiratory depression ensues
Side Effects:	Respiratory depression Drowsiness
Dosage:	1–4 g
Routes:	IV Intramuscular
Pediatric Dosage:	Not indicated

Mannitol (Osmotrol®)

Class:	Osmotic diuretic
Actions:	Decreases cellular edema Increases urinary output
Indications:	Acute cerebral edema Blood transfusion reactions
Contraindications:	Pulmonary edema Patients who are dehydrated Hypersensitivity to the drug
Precautions:	Rapid administration can cause circulatory overload Crystallization of the drug can occur at lower temperatures An in-line filter should be used

Side Effects:	Pulmonary congestion
	Sodium depletion
	Transient volume overload
Dosage:	0.5–1 g/kg
Route:	IV
Pediatric Dosage:	0.25–0.5 g/kg IV over 60 minutes

Meperidine (Demerol®)

Class:	Narcotic
Actions:	Central nervous system depressant
	Decreases sensitivity to pain
Indications:	Severe pain
Contraindications:	Patients receiving monoamine oxidase inhibitors
	Undiagnosed abdominal pain
	Patients with history of hypersensitivity to the drug
Precautions:	Respiratory depression (Narcan should be available)
	Hypotension
	Nausea
Side Effects:	Dizziness
	Altered level of consciousness
Dosage:	IV
	25–50 mg
	Intramuscular
	50–100 mg
Routes:	IV
	Intramuscular
Pediatric Dosage:	1 mg/kg

Metaproterenol (Alupent®)

Class:	Sympathomimetic (β_2 selective)
Actions:	Bronchodilation
	Increases heart rate

Indications:	Bronchial asthma Reversible bronchospasm associated with chronic bronchitis and emphysema
Contraindications:	Patients with cardiac dysrhythmias or significant tachycardia
Precautions:	Blood pressure, pulse, and EKG must be constantly monitored; occasional nausea and vomiting reported
Side Effects:	Palpitations, anxiety, headache, nausea, vomiting, dizziness, and tremor
Dosage:	*Metered Dose Inhaler* 2–3 inhalations; can be repeated in 3–4 hours if required *Small-Volume Nebulizer* 0.2–0.3 ml diluted in 2–3 ml normal saline administered over 5–15 minutes
Route:	Inhalation only
Pediatric Dosage:	0.05–0.3 ml in 4 ml normal saline

Metaraminol (Aramine®)

Class:	Sympathomimetic (indirect acting)
Actions:	Causes release of endogenous stores of norepinephrine Increases cardiac contractile force Increases cardiac rate Causes peripheral vasoconstriction
Indication:	Cardiogenic shock
Contraindications:	Hypotensive states due to hypovolemia
Precautions:	Constant monitoring of blood pressure is essential Not effective in catecholamine-depleted patients
Side Effects:	Palpitations, tachycardia, and PVCs Hypertension, tremor, and dizziness
Dosage:	200 mg should be placed in 500 ml of D_5W; this gives a concentration of 0.4 mg/ml, which should be slowly infused and titrated to blood pressure response

Route: IV drip only

Pediatric Dosage: Safety in children has not been established

---

Methylprednisolone (Solu-Medrol®)

Class: Steroid

Actions: Anti-inflammatory
                                Suppresses immune response (especially in allergic reactions)

Indications: Severe anaphylaxis
                                Possibly effective as an adjunctive agent in the management of spinal cord injury

Contraindications: None in the emergency setting

Precautions: Must be reconstituted and used promptly
                                Onset of action may be 2–6 hours and thus should not be expected to be of use in the critical first hour following an anaphylactic reaction

Side Effects: GI bleeding
                                Prolonged wound healing
                                Suppression of natural steroids

Dosage: 125–250 mg

Routes: IV
                                Intramuscular

Pediatric Dosage: 30 μg/kg

Metoprolol (Lopressor®)

Class: Sympathetic blocker (β_2 selective)

Action: Selectively block β_2 adrenergic receptors (cardioprotective)

Indications: Suspected or definite acute myocardial infarction in patients who are hemodynamically stable

Contraindications: Heart rate less than 45 beats per minute
                                Heart block
                                Shock
                                History of asthma
                                History of bronchospastic disease

Precautions:	Blood pressure, pulse and EKG must be constantly monitored
	Atropine and isoproterenol should be available
Side Effects:	Bradycardia
	Heart block
	Congestive heart failure
	Depression
	Bronchospasm
Dosage:	Initial bolus of 5 mg slow IV injection
	May repeat in 5 minutes if vital signs are stable
	May repeat in 10 minutes if vital signs are stable
Route:	Slow IV bolus
Pediatric Dosage:	Safety in children has not been established

Morphine

Class:	Narcotic
Actions:	Central nervous system depressant
	Causes peripheral vasodilation
	Decreases sensitivity to pain
Indications:	Severe pain
	Pulmonary edema
Contraindications:	Head injury
	Volume depletion
	Undiagnosed abdominal pain
	Patients with history of hypersensitivity to the drug
Precautions:	Respiratory depression (Narcan® should be available)
	Hypotension
	Nausea
Side Effects:	Dizziness
	Altered level of consciousness
Dosage:	IV
	2–5 mg followed by 2 mg every few minutes until the pain is relieved or until respiratory depression ensues

Intramuscular
5–15 mg based on patient weight

Routes: IV
                       Intramuscular

Pediatric Dosage: 0.1–0.2 mg/kg IV

Nalbuphine (Nubain®)

Class: Synthetic analgesic

Actions: Central nervous system depressant
                        Decreases sensitivity to pain

Indications: Moderate to severe pain

Contraindication: Patients with a history of hypersensitivity to the drug

Precautions: Use with caution in patients with impaired respiratory function
                        Respiratory depression (Narcan® should be available)
                        Patients dependent on narcotics may experience symptoms of withdrawal
                        Nausea

Side Effects: Dizziness
                        Altered level of consciousness

Dosage: 5–10 mg

Routes: IV
                        Intramuscular

Pediatric Dosage: Rarely used

Naloxone (Narcan®)

Class: Narcotic antagonist

Action: Reverses effects of narcotics

Indications: Narcotic overdoses including the following:

                    morphine   methadone
                    Dilaudid   heroin

fentanyl   Percodan
Demerol   Tylox
Paregoric

Synthetic analgesic overdoses including the following:

Nubain   Talwin
Stadol   Darvon

Alcoholic coma
To rule out narcotics in coma of unknown origin

Contraindication:	Patients with a history of hypersensitivity to the drug
Precautions:	Should be administered with caution to patients dependent on narcotics as it may cause withdrawal effects
	Short-acting, should be augmented every 5 minutes
Side Effects:	None
Dosage:	1–2 mg
Routes:	IV
	Intramuscular
	Endotracheal
Pediatric Dosage:	0.01–0.1 mg/kg

Nifedipine (Procardia®)

Class:	Calcium channel blocker
Action:	Relaxes smooth muscle causing arteriolar vasodilation
	Decreases peripheral vascular resistance
Indications:	Severe hypertension
	Angina pectoris
Contraindications:	Known hypersensitivity to the drug
	Hypotension
Precautions:	Blood pressure should be constantly monitored
	May worsen congestive heart failure

	Nifedipine should not be administered to patients receiving intravenous beta blockers
Side Effects:	Dizziness, flushing, nausea, headache, and weakness
Dosage:	10 mg sublingually; puncture the capsule several times with a needle and place it under the patient's tongue and have them withdraw the liquid medication
Route:	Oral Sublingual
Pediatric Dosage:	0.25–0.5 mg/kg

Nitroglycerin (Nitrostat®)

Class:	Antianginal
Actions:	Smooth-muscle relaxant Reduces cardiac work Dilates coronary arteries Dilates systemic arteries
Indications:	Angina pectoris Chest pain associated with myocardial infarction
Contraindications:	Children younger than 12 years of age Hypotension
Precautions:	Constantly monitor blood pressure Syncope Drug must be protected from light Expires quickly once bottle is opened
Side Effects:	Headache Dizziness Hypotension
Dosage:	1 tablet repeated up to 3 times
Route:	Sublingual
Pediatric Dosage:	Not indicated

Nitroglycerin Spray (Nitrolingual Spray)

Class:	Antianginal

Actions:	Smooth-muscle relaxant Decreases cardiac work Dilates coronary arteries Dilates systemic arteries
Indications:	Angina pectoris Chest pain associated with myocardial infarction
Contraindications:	Hypotension
Precautions:	Constantly monitor vital signs Syncope can occur
Side Effects:	Dizziness Hypotension Headache
Dosage:	One spray administered under the tongue; may be repeated in 10–15 minutes; no more than three sprays in a 15-minute period; spray should not be inhaled
Route:	Sprayed under tongue on mucous membrane
Pediatric Dosage:	Not indicated

Nitropaste (Nitro-Bid®)

Class:	Antianginal
Actions:	Smooth-muscle relaxant Decreases cardiac work Dilates coronary arteries Dilates systemic arteries
Indications:	Angina pectoris Chest pain associated with myocardial infarction
Contraindications:	Children younger than 12 years of age Hypotension
Precautions:	Constantly monitor blood pressure Syncope Drug must be protected from light Expires quickly once bottle is opened
Side Effects:	Dizziness Hypotension
Dosage:	1/2 to 3/4 inches

Route:	Topical
Pediatric Dosage:	Not indicated

Nitrous Oxide (Nitronox®)

Class:	Gas
Action:	Central nervous system depressant
Indications:	Pain of musculoskeletal origin, particularly fractures
	Burns
	Suspected ischemic chest pain
	States of severe anxiety including hyperventilation
Contraindications:	Patients who cannot comprehend verbal instructions
	Patients intoxicated with alcohol or drugs
	Head-injury patients who exhibit an altered mental status
	COPD (increased oxygen concentration may cause respiratory depression)
	Thoracic injury suspicious for pneumothorax
	Abdominal pain and distension suggestive of bowel obstruction
Precautions:	Use only in well-ventilated area
	Gas-scavenging system is recommended
	May not operate properly at low temperatures
Side Effects:	Headache, dizziness, giddiness, nausea, and vomiting
Dosage:	Self-administered only using fixed 50% nitrous oxide/50% oxygen blender
Route:	Inhalation only
Pediatric Dosage:	Self-administered only

Norepinephrine (Levophed®)

Class:	Sympathomimetic
Action:	Causes peripheral vasoconstriction

Indications:	Hypotension refractory to other sympatho-mimetics Neurogenic shock
Contraindications:	Hypotensive states due to hypovolemia
Precautions:	Can be deactivated by alkaline solutions Constant monitoring of blood pressure is essential
Side Effects:	Palpitations Hypertension Local venous irritation
Dosages:	2–12 μg/minute *Method* 8 mg should be placed in 500 ml of D_5W, giving a concentration of 16 μg/ml
Route:	IV drip only
Pediatric Dosage:	0.01–0.5 μg/kg/minute (rarely used)

Oxygen

Class:	Gas
Action:	Necessary for cellular metabolism
Indications:	Hypoxia
Contraindications:	None
Precautions:	Use cautiously in patients with COPD Humidify when providing high-flow rates
Side Effects:	Drying of mucous membranes
Dosage:	*Cardiac Arrest* 100% *COPD* 24–35%
Route:	Inhalation
Pediatric Dosage:	24–100% as required

Oxytocin (Pitocin®)

Class:	Hormone (oxytocic)

Actions:	Causes uterine contraction Causes lactation Slows postpartum vaginal bleeding
Indication:	Postpartum vaginal bleeding
Contraindications:	Any condition other than postpartum bleeding Cesarean section
Precautions:	Essential to assure that the placenta has delivered and that there is not another fetus present before administering oxytocin Overdosage can cause uterine rupture Hypertension
Side Effects:	Anaphylaxis Cardiac arrhythmias
Dosage:	IV 10–20 units in 500 ml of D_5W administered according to uterine response *Intramuscular* 3–10 units
Routes:	IV drip Intramuscular
Pediatric Dosage:	Not indicated

Phenobarbital

Class:	Barbiturate
Actions:	Suppresses spread of seizure activity through the motor cortex Central nervous system depressant
Indications:	Major motor seizures Status epilepticus Acute anxiety states
Contraindication:	History of hypersensitivity to the drug
Precautions:	Respiratory depression Hypotension Can cause hyperactivity in children Extravasation may cause tissue necrosis

Side Effects:	Drowsiness Children may become hyperactive
Dosage:	100–250 mg
Route:	IV Intramuscular
Pediatric Dosage:	10 mg/kg

Phenytoin (Dilantin®)

Class:	Anticonvulsant
Action:	Inhibits spread of seizure activity through motor cortex Antiarrhythmic
Indications:	Major motor seizures Status epilepticus Arrhythmias due to digitalis toxicity
Contraindications:	Any arrhythmia except those due to digitalis toxicity Patients with history of hypersensitivity to the drug
Precautions:	Should not be administered with sugar solutions Hypotension EKG monitoring during administration is essential
Side Effects:	Local venous irritation Central nervous system depression
Dosages:	*Status Epilepticus* 150–250 mg (10–15 mg/kg) not to exceed 50 mg/minute *Digitalis Toxicity* 100 mg over 5 minutes until the arrhythmia is suppressed or until symptoms of central nervous system depression occur
Route:	IV (dilute with saline)
Pediatric Dosages:	*Status Epilepticus* 8–10 mg/kg IV *Digitalis Toxicity* 3–5 mg/kg IV over 10 minutes

Physostigmine (Antilirium®)

Class:	Cholinesterase inhibitor
Actions:	Inhibits cholinesterase Potentiates acetylcholine
Indications:	Tricyclic overdoses including the following:

Tofranil   Elavil
Norpramin   Adapin
Sinequan

Atropine/Belladonna overdoses

Contraindications:	Asthma and COPD Gangrene Diabetics Cardiovascular disease
Precautions:	Monitor for bronchospasm and laryngospasm Seizures
Side Effects:	Excessive salivation Bradycardia Emesis
Dosage:	0.5–2.0 mg
Route:	IV
Pediatric Dosage:	0.5–1.0 mg over 5 minutes

Pralidoxime (2-PAM) (Protopam®)

Class:	Cholinesterase reactivator
Actions:	Reactivates cholinesterase in cases of organo-phosphate poisoning Deactivates certain organophosphates by direct chemical reaction
Indications:	Severe organophosphate poisoning as character-ized by muscle twitching, respiratory depres-sion, and paralysis
Contraindications:	Poisonings due to inorganic phosphates Poisonings other than organophosphates

Precautions:	Always assure safety and protection of rescue personnel
	Laryngospasm, tachycardia, and muscle rigidity have occurred following rapid administration
	Should only follow atropinization
Side Effects:	Excitement
	Manic behavior
Dosage:	1 g in 250–500 ml of normal saline infused over 30 minutes
Route:	IV drip
Pediatric Dosage:	20–40 mg/kg by the same method

Procainamide (Pronestyl®)

Class:	Antiarrhythmic
Actions:	Slows conduction through myocardium
	Elevates ventricular fibrillation threshold
	Suppresses ventricular ectopic activity
Indications:	PVCs refractory to lidocaine
	Ventricular tachycardia refractory to lidocaine
Contraindications:	High-degree heart blocks
	PVCs in conjunction with bradycardia
Precautions:	Dosage should not exceed 1 g
	Monitor for central nervous system toxicity
Side Effects:	Anxiety
	Nausea
	Convulsions
	Widening of QRS
Dosage:	*Initial*
	20 mg/minute until
	Arrhythmia abolished
	Hypotension ensues
	QRS widened by 50% of original width
	Total of 1 g has been given
	Maintenance
	1–4 mg/minute

Routes: Slow IV bolus
                         IV drip

Pediatric Dosage: Rarely used

| **Promethazine (Phenergan®)** |

Class: Antihistamine (H_1 antagonist)

Actions: Mild anticholinergic activity
                         Antiemetic
                         Potentiates actions of analgesics

Indications: Nausea and vomiting
                         Motion sickness
                         To potentiate the effects of analgesics

Contraindications: Comatose states
                         Patients who have received a large amount of de-
                         pressants

Precaution: Avoid accidental intra-arterial injection

Side Effects: May impair mental and physical ability
                         Drowsiness

Dosage: 25 mg

Route: IV

Pediatric Dosage: 0.5 mg/kg

| **Propranolol (Inderal®)** |

Class: Sympathetic blocker

Action: Nonselectively blocks β-adrenergic receptors

Indications: Ventricular tachyarrhythmias refractory to lido-
                         caine
                         Ventricular fibrillation refractory to lidocaine
                         Tachyarrhythmias due to digitalis toxicity

Contraindications: Asthmatics
                         Patients dependent on sympathetic agonists
                         COPD

Precautions:	Should not be given concurrently with verapamil Atropine and isoproterenol should be readily available
Side Effects:	Bradycardia Heart blocks Congestive heart failure Bronchospasm
Dosage:	1–3 mg diluted in 10–30 ml of D_5W given slowly IV
Route:	Slow IV bolus
Pediatric Dosage:	0.01 mg/kg

Racemic Epinephrine (MicroNEFRIN®)

Class:	Sympathomimetic
Actions:	Bronchodilation Increases heart rate Increases cardiac contractile force
Indications:	Croup (laryngotracheobronchitis)
Contraindications:	Epiglottitis Hypersensitivity to the drug
Precautions:	Vital signs should be constantly monitored Should be used only once
Side Effects:	Palpitations Anxiety Headache
Dosage:	0.5 ml of a 2.25% solution in 2.5 ml normal saline
Route:	Inhalation only (small-volume nebulizer)
Pediatric Dosage:	0.25–0.5 ml of a 2.25% solution in 4 ml normal saline

---

Sodium Bicarbonate

Class:	Alkalinizing agent

Actions:	Combines with excessive acids to form a weak volatile acid
	Increases pH
Indications:	Late in the management of cardiac arrest, if at all
	Tricyclic antidepressant overdose
	Severe acidosis refractory to hyperventilation
Contraindication:	Alkalotic states
Precautions:	Correct dosage is essential to avoid overcompensation of pH
	Can deactivate catecholamines
	Can precipitate with calcium
	Delivers large sodium load
Side Effects:	Alkalosis
Dosage:	1 mEq/kg initially followed by 1/2 mEq/kg every 10 minutes as indicated by blood gas studies
Route:	IV
Pediatric Dosage:	1 mEq/kg initially followed by 1/2 mEq/kg every 10 minutes

---

Sodium Nitroprusside (Nipride®, Nitropress®)

Class:	Potent vasodilator
Actions:	Peripheral arterial and venous vasodilator
	Decreases blood pressure
	Increases cardiac output in CHF
Indications:	Hypertensive emergency
Contraindications:	None when used in the management of life-threatening emergency
Precautions:	Bottle must be wrapped in foil to protect from light
	Should not be administered to children or pregnant women in the prehospital setting
	Reduce the dosage in elderly patients
	Blood pressure, pulse, and EKG must be diligently monitored
Side Effects:	Nausea, retching, vomiting, palpitations, diaphoresis, tachycardia, and dizziness; side effects often diminish as dosage is reduced

Dosage:	0.5 μg/kg/minute
Route:	IV infusion only
Pediatric Dosage:	Not indicated in prehospital setting

Succinylcholine (Anectine®)

Class:	Neuromuscular blocking agent (depolarizing)
Action:	Skeletal muscle relaxant Paralyzes skeletal muscles including respiratory muscles
Indications:	To achieve paralysis to facilitate endotracheal intubation
Contraindications:	Patients with known hypersensitivity to the drug
Precautions:	Should not be administered unless persons skilled in endotracheal intubation are present Endotracheal intubation equipment must be available Oxygen equipment and emergency resuscitative drugs must be available Paralysis occurs within 1 minute and lasts for approximately 8 minutes
Side Effects:	Prolonged paralysis Hypotension Bradycardia
Dosage:	1 mg/kg (20–80 mg in an adult)
Route:	IV
Pediatric Dosage:	1 mg/kg

Terbutaline (Brethine®)

Class:	Sympathomimetic
Action:	Bronchodilator Increases heart rate
Indications:	Bronchial asthma Reversible bronchospasm associated with COPD

Contraindications:	Patients with known hypersensitivity to the drug
Precautions:	Blood pressure, pulse, and EKG must be constantly monitored
Side Effects:	Palpitations, tachycardia, and PVCs
	Anxiety, tremor, and headache
Dosage:	*Metered-Dose Inhaler*
	Two inhalations, 1 minute apart
	Subcutaneous Injection
	0.25 mg; may be repeated in 15–30 minutes
Route:	Inhalation
	Subcutaneous injection
Pediatric Dosage:	0.01 mg/kg subcutaneously

Thiamine (Vitamin B₁)

Class:	Vitamin
Action:	Allows normal breakdown of glucose
Indications:	Coma of unknown origin
	Alcoholism
	Delirium tremens
Contraindications:	None in the emergency setting
Precautions:	Rare anaphylactic reactions have been reported
Side Effects:	Rare, if any
Dosage:	100 mg
Route:	IV
	Intramuscular
Pediatric Dosage:	Rarely indicated

Verapamil (Isoptin®) (Calan®)

Class:	Calcium channel blocker
Action:	Slows conduction through the AV node
	Inhibits reentry during PSVT
	Decreases rate of ventricular response
	Decreases myocardial oxygen demand

Indications: PSVT

Contraindications: Heart block
                            Conduction system disturbances

Precautions: Should not be used in patients receiving intrave-
                                nous β-blockers
                            Hypotension

Side Effects: Nausea, vomiting, hypotension, and dizziness

Dosage: 2.5–5 mg; may be repeated after 20–30 minutes if
                                PSVT does not convert

Route: Intravenous

Pediatric Dosage: *0–1 Year*
                            0.1–0.2 mg/kg (maximum of 2.0 mg) adminis-
                            tered slowly
                            1–15 years
                            0.1–0.3 mg/kg (maximum of 5.0 mg) adminis-
                            tered slowly

APPENDIX B

EMERGENCY IV FLUIDS

Plasma Protein Fraction (Plasmanate®)

Class:	Protein colloid
Action:	Plasma volume expander
Indication:	Hypovolemic states (especially burn shock)
Contraindications:	None when used in the management of life-threatening situations
Precautions:	Hypertension Short shelf life
Side Effects:	Edema
Dosage:	Dosage should be titrated according to patient's hemodynamic response; follow accepted resuscitation formulas in the management of burn shock
Route:	IV infusion
Pediatric Dosage:	Same as adult

TABLE B–1 Approximate Ionic Concentrations (mEq/l) and Calories per Liter

	Ionic Concentrations (mEq/l)					Calories per liter	Osmolarity[a] (mOsm/l)	pH Range
	Sodium	Potassium	Calcium	Chloride	Lactate			
5% Dextrose Injection, USP	0	0	0	0	0	170	252	3.5–6.5
10% Dextrose Injection, USP	0	0	0	0	0	340	505	3.5–6.5
0.9% Sodium Chloride Injection, USP	154	0	0	154	0	0	308	4.5–7.0
Sodium Lactate Injection, USP (M/6 Sodium Lactate)	167	0	0	0	167	54	334	6.0–7.3
2.5% Dextrose & 0.45% Sodium Chloride Injection, USP	77	0	0	77	0	85	280	3.5–6.0
5% Dextrose & 0.2% Sodium Chloride Injection, USP	34	0	0	34	0	170	321	3.5–6.0
5% Dextrose & 0.33% Sodium Chloride Injection, USP	56	0	0	56	0	170	365	3.5–6.0
5% Dextrose & 0.45% Sodium Chloride Injection, USP	77	0	0	77	0	170	406	3.5–6.0
5% Dextrose & 0.9% Sodium Chloride Injection, USP	154	0	0	154	0	170	560	3.5–6.0
10% Dextrose & 0.9% Sodium Chloride Injection, USP	154	0	0	154	0	340	813	3.5–6.0
Ringer's Injection, USP	147.5	4	4.5	156	0	0	309	5.0–7.5
Lactated Ringer's Injection, USP	130	4	3	109	28	9	273	6.0–7.5
5% Dextrose in Ringer's Injection	147.5	4	4.5	156	0	170	561	3.5–6.5
Lactated Ringer's with 5% Dextrose	130	4	3	109	28	180	525	4.0–6.5

[a]Normal physiological isotonicity range is approximately 280–310 mOsm/l. Administration of substantially hypotonic solutions may cause hemolysis and administration of substantially hypertonic solutions may cause vein damage.
(Adapted with permission from Travenol Laboratories, Inc., Deerfield, Illinois)

Dextran

Class:	Imitation protein (sugar) colloid
Action:	Plasma volume expander
Indication:	Hypovolemic shock
Contraindications:	Patients with known hypersensitivity to the drug Patients receiving anticoagulants
Precautions:	Severe anaphylactic reactions have been known to occur Monitor for circulatory overload Can impede accurate blood typing as dextran molecule coats the erythrocytes; Draw tube of blood for blood typing before administering Dextran
Side Effects:	Nausea Vomiting
Dosage:	Dosage should be titrated according to patient's hemodynamic response
Route:	IV infusion
Pediatric Dosage:	Same as adult

Hetastarch (Hespan®)

Class:	Artificial colloid
Action:	Plasma volume expander
Indication:	Hypovolemic shock
Contraindication:	Patients receiving anticoagulants
Precautions:	Monitor for circulatory overload Large volumes of hetastarch may alter the coagulation mechanism
Side Effects:	Nausea Vomiting
Dosage:	Dosage should be titrated according to patient's hemodynamic response
Route:	IV infusion
Pediatric Dosage:	Safety in children has not been established

Lactated Ringer's

Class:	Isotonic crystalloid
Action:	Approximates the electrolyte concentration of the blood
Indication:	Hypovolemic shock
Contraindications:	Congestive heart failure Renal failure
Precaution:	Monitor for circulatory overload
Side Effects:	Rare
Dosage:	*Hypovolemic Shock (systolic less than 90 mmHg)* Infuse "wide open" until a systolic of 100 mmHg is attained; once a systolic of 100 mmHg has been attained, infusion should be slowed to 100 ml/hr *Other* As indicated by the patient condition and situation being treated
Route:	IV infusion
Pediatric Dosage:	20 ml/kg repeated as required based on hemodynamic response

5% Dextrose in water (D₅W)

Class:	Sugar solution
Action:	Glucose nutrient solution
Indications:	IV access for emergency drugs For dilution of concentrated drugs for IV infusion
Contraindication:	Should not be used as a fluid replacement for hypovolemic states
Precautions:	Monitor for circulatory overload Draw tube of blood before administering to diabetics
Side Effects:	Rare
Dosage:	Generally administered TKO

Route: IV infusion

Pediatric Dosage: Same as adult

| **10% Dextrose in water (D₁₀W)** |

Class: Hypertonic sugar solution

Action: Replaces blood glucose

Indications: Hypoglycemia
                        Neonatal resuscitation

Contraindications: Should not be used as fluid replacement for hypovolemic states

Precautions: Monitor for circulatory overload
                        Draw tube of blood before administering $D_{10}W$ to diabetics

Side Effects: Rare

Dosage: Dependent on patient condition and condition being treated

Route: IV infusion

Pediatric Dosage: Same as adult

| **0.9% Sodium Chloride (Normal Saline)** |

Class: Isotonic electrolyte

Action: Fluid and sodium replacement

Indication: Heat-related problems (heat exhaustion and heat stroke)
                        Freshwater drowning
                        Hypovolemia
                        Diabetic ketoacidosis

Contraindications: Congestive heart failure

Precautions: Electrolyte depletion (K^+, Mg^{++}, Ca^{++}, among others) can occur following administration of large amounts of normal saline

Side Effects: Thirst

Dosage:	Dependent on patient condition and situation being treated; in freshwater drowning and heat emergencies, the administration is usually rapid
Route:	IV infusion
Pediatric Dosage:	Dose is dependent on patient size and condition

0.45% Sodium Chloride (½ Normal Saline)

Class:	Hypotonic electrolyte
Action:	Slow rehydration
Indications:	Patients with diminished renal or cardiovascular function for which rapid rehydration is not indicated
Contraindications:	Cases in which rapid rehydration is indicated
Precautions:	Electrolyte depletion can occur following administration of large amounts of 1/2 normal saline
Side Effects:	Rare
Dosage:	Dependent on patient condition and situation being treated
Route:	IV infusion
Pediatric Dosage:	Dose is based on patient size and condition

5% Dextrose in 0.9% Sodium Chloride (D₅NS)

Class:	Hypertonic sugar and electrolyte solution
Actions:	Provides electrolyte and sugar replacement
Indications:	Heat-related disorders Freshwater drowning Hypovolemia Peritonitis
Contraindications:	Should not be administered to patients with impaired renal or cardiovascular function
Precaution:	Draw tube of blood before administering to diabetics

Side Effects:	Rare
Dosage:	Dependent on patient condition and situation being treated
Route:	IV infusion
Pediatric Dosage:	Dose is dependent on patient size and condition

---

5% Dextrose in 0.45% of Sodium Chloride (D₅ ½ NS)

Class:	Slightly hypertonic sugar and electrolyte solution
Action:	Provides electrolyte and sugar replacement
Indications:	Heat exhaustion Diabetic disorders For use as a TKO solution in patients with impaired renal or cardiovascular function
Contraindications:	Situations in which rapid fluid replacement is indicated
Precaution:	Draw tube of blood before administering to diabetics
Side Effects:	Rare
Dosage:	Dependent on patient condition and situation being treated
Route:	IV infusion
Pediatric Dosage:	Dose is dependent on patient size and condition

---

5% Dextrose in lactated ringer's (D₅LR)

Class:	Hypertonic sugar and electrolyte solution
Actions:	Provides electrolyte and sugar replacement
Indications:	Hypovolemic shock Hemorrhagic shock Certain cases of acidosis
Contraindications:	Should not be administered to patients with decreased renal or cardiovascular function

Precautions: Monitor for signs of circulatory overload
                          Draw tube of blood before administering to dia-
                          betics

Side Effects: Rare

Dosage: Dependent on patient condition and situation
                          being treated

Route: IV infusion

Pediatric Dosage: Dose is dependent on patient size and condition

APPENDIX C

ACLS TREATMENT ALGORITHMS

Ventricular Fibrillation and Pulseless Ventricular Tachycardia[a]

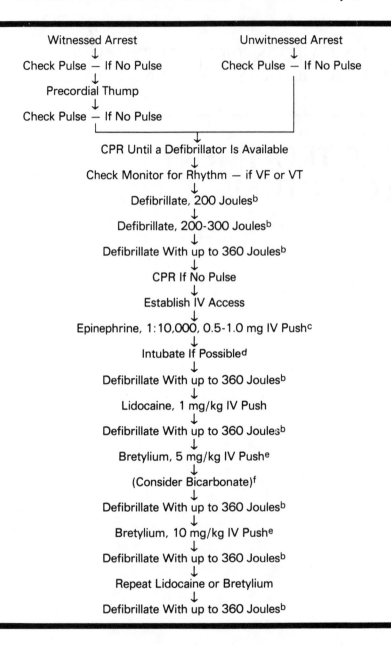

Witnessed Arrest
↓
Check Pulse — If No Pulse
↓
Precordial Thump
↓
Check Pulse — If No Pulse

Unwitnessed Arrest
↓
Check Pulse — If No Pulse

CPR Until a Defibrillator Is Available
↓
Check Monitor for Rhythm — if VF or VT
↓
Defibrillate, 200 Joules[b]
↓
Defibrillate, 200-300 Joules[b]
↓
Defibrillate With up to 360 Joules[b]
↓
CPR If No Pulse
↓
Establish IV Access
↓
Epinephrine, 1:10,000, 0.5-1.0 mg IV Push[c]
↓
Intubate If Possible[d]
↓
Defibrillate With up to 360 Joules[b]
↓
Lidocaine, 1 mg/kg IV Push
↓
Defibrillate With up to 360 Joules[b]
↓
Bretylium, 5 mg/kg IV Push[e]
↓
(Consider Bicarbonate)[f]
↓
Defibrillate With up to 360 Joules[b]
↓
Bretylium, 10 mg/kg IV Push[e]
↓
Defibrillate With up to 360 Joules[b]
↓
Repeat Lidocaine or Bretylium
↓
Defibrillate With up to 360 Joules[b]

Ventricular Fibrillation and Pulseless Ventricular Tachycardia[a]

Notes To Figure A

[a]Pulseless VT should be treated identically to VF.

[b]Check pulse and rhythm after each shock. If VF recurs after transiently converting (rather than persists without ever converting), use whatever energy level has previously been successful for defibrillation.

[c]Epinephrine should be repeated every five minutes.

[d]Intubation is preferable. It can be accompanied simultaneously with other techniques, then the earlier the better. However, defibrillation and epinephrine are more important initially if the patient can be ventilated without intubation.

[e]Some may prefer repeated doses of lidocaine, which may be given in 0.5-mg/kg boluses every eight minutes to a total dose of 3 mg/kg.

[f]Value of sodium bicarbonate is questionable during cardiac arrest, and it is not recommended for routine cardiac arrest sequence. Consideration of its use in a dose of 1 mEq/kg is appropriate at this point. Half of original dose may be repeated every ten minutes if it is used.

Asystole

If Rhythm Is Unclear and Possibly Ventricular
Fibrillation, Defibrillate as for VF. If Asystole is Present[a]
↓
Continue CPR
↓
Establish IV Access
↓
Epinephrine, 1:10,000, 0.5 -1.0 mg IV Push[b]
↓
Intubate When Possible[c]
↓
Atropine, 1.0 mg IV Push (Repeated in 5 min)
↓
(Consider Bicarbonate)[d]
↓
Consider Pacing

[a]Asystole should be confirmed in two leads.
[b]Epinephrine should be repeated every five minutes.
[c]Intubation is preferable; if it can be accompanied simultaneously with other techniques, then the earlier the better. However, cardiopulmonary resuscitation (CPR) and use of epinephrine are more important initially if patient can be ventilated without intubation. (Endotracheal epinephrine may be used.)
[d]Value of sodium bicarbonate is questionable during cardiac arrest, and it is not recommended for the routine cardiac arrest sequence. Consideration of its use in a dose of 1 mEq/kg is appropriate at this point. Half of original dose may be repeated every ten minutes if it is used.

Electromechanical Dissociation

Continue CPR
↓
Establish IV Access
↓
Epinephrine, 1:10,000, 0.5 -1.0 mg IV Push[a]
↓
Intubate When Possible[b]
↓
(Consider Bicarbonate)[c]
↓
Consider Hypovolemia,
Cardiac Tamponade,
Tension Pneumothorax,
Hypoxemia,
Acidosis,
Pulmonary Embolism

[a]Epinephrine should be repeated every five minutes.

[b]Intubation is preferable. If it can be accomplished simultaneously with other techniques, then the earlier the better. However, epinephrine is more important initially if the patient can be ventilated without intubation.

[c]Value of sodium bicarbonate is questionable during cardiac arrest, and it is not recommended for routine cardiac arrest sequence. Consideration of its use in a dose of 1 mEq/kg is appropriate at this point. Half of original dose may be repeated every ten minutes if it is used.

Sustained Ventricular Tachycardia

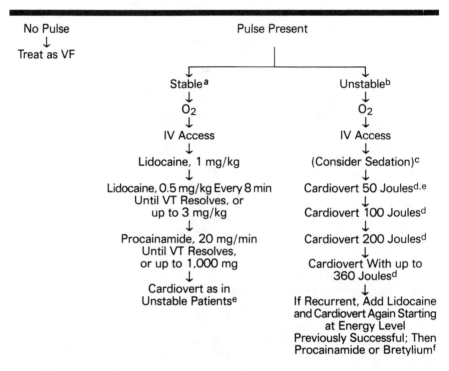

No Pulse
↓
Treat as VF

Pulse Present

Stable[a]
↓
O₂
↓
IV Access
↓
Lidocaine, 1 mg/kg
↓
Lidocaine, 0.5 mg/kg Every 8 min
Until VT Resolves, or
up to 3 mg/kg
↓
Procainamide, 20 mg/min
Until VT Resolves,
or up to 1,000 mg
↓
Cardiovert as in
Unstable Patients[e]

Unstable[b]
↓
O₂
↓
IV Access
↓
(Consider Sedation)[c]
↓
Cardiovert 50 Joules[d,e]
↓
Cardiovert 100 Joules[d]
↓
Cardiovert 200 Joules[d]
↓
Cardiovert With up to
360 Joules[d]
↓
If Recurrent, Add Lidocaine
and Cardiovert Again Starting
at Energy Level
Previously Successful; Then
Procainamide or Bretylium[f]

[a]If patient becomes unstable (see footnote b for definition) at any time, move to "Unstable" arm of algorithm.

[b]Unstable indicates symptoms (e.g., chest pain or dyspnea), hypotension (systolic blood pressure <90 mmHg), congestive heart failure, ischemia, or infarction.

[c]Sedation should be considered for all patients, including those defined in footnote b as unstable, except those who are hemodynamically unstable (e.g., hypotensive, in pulmonary edema, or unconscious).

[d]If hypotension, pulmonary edema, or unconsciousness is present, unsynchronized cardioversion should be done to avoid delay associated with synchronization.

[e]In the absence of hypotension, pulmonary edema, or unconsciousness, a precordial thump may be employed prior to cardioversion.

[f]Once VT has resolved, begin intravenous (IV) infusion of antiarrhythmic agent that has aided resolution of VT. If hypotension, pulmonary edema, or unconsciousness is present, use lidocaine if cardioversion alone is unsuccessful, followed by bretylium. In all other patients, recommended order of therapy is lidocaine, procainamide, and then bretylium.

Bradycardia

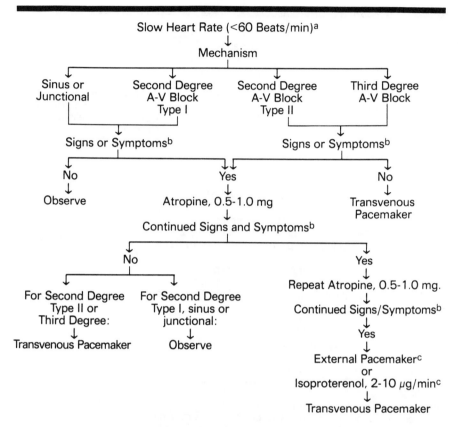

Slow Heart Rate (<60 Beats/min)ᵃ
↓
Mechanism

Sinus or Junctional | Second Degree A-V Block Type I | Second Degree A-V Block Type II | Third Degree A-V Block

Signs or Symptomsᵇ   Signs or Symptomsᵇ

No → Observe

Yes → Atropine, 0.5-1.0 mg
↓
Continued Signs and Symptomsᵇ

No → Transvenous Pacemaker

No:
For Second Degree Type II or Third Degree: → Transvenous Pacemaker
For Second Degree Type I, sinus or junctional: → Observe

Yes:
Repeat Atropine, 0.5-1.0 mg.
↓
Continued Signs/Symptomsᵇ
↓
Yes
↓
External Pacemakerᶜ
or
Isoproterenol, 2-10 µg/minᶜ
↓
Transvenous Pacemaker

ᵃA solitary chest thump or cough may stimulate cardiac electrical activity and result in improved cardiac output and may be used at this point.

ᵇHypotension (blood pressure < 90 mmHg), premature ventricular contractions, altered mental status or symptoms (e.g., chest pain or dyspnea), ischemia, or infarction.

ᶜTemporizing therapy.

Ventricular Ectopy

Assess for Need for
Acute Suppressive Therapy
↓

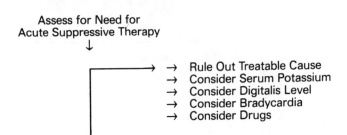

→ → Rule Out Treatable Cause
→ Consider Serum Potassium
→ Consider Digitalis Level
→ Consider Bradycardia
→ Consider Drugs

Lidocaine, 1 mg/kg[a]
↓
If Not Suppressed,
Repeat Lidocaine, 0.5 mg/kg Every 2-5 min,
Until No Ectopy, or up to 3 mg/kg Given
↓
If Not Suppressed,
Procainamide 20 mg/min
Until No Ectopy, or up to 1,000 mg Given
↓
If Not Suppressed,
and Not Contraindicated,
Bretylium, 5-10 mg/kg Over 8-10 min
↓
If Not Suppressed,
Consider Overdrive Pacing

Once Ectopy Resolved, Maintain as Follows:
After Lidocaine, 1 mg/kg...Lidocaine Drip, 2 mg/min
After Lidocaine, 1-2 mg/kg...Lidocaine Drip, 3 mg/min
After Lidocaine, 2-3 mg/kg...Lidocaine Drip, 4 mg/min
After Procainamide...Procainamide drip, 1-4 mg/min (Check Blood Level)
After Bretylium...Bretylium Drip, 2 mg/min

[a]Reduce lidocaine dosage by 50% in patients >70 years of age.

PSVT

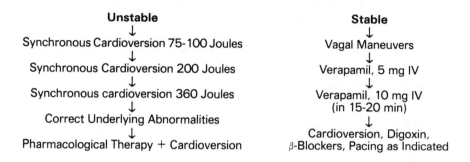

Unstable	Stable
↓	↓
Synchronous Cardioversion 75-100 Joules	Vagal Maneuvers
↓	↓
Synchronous Cardioversion 200 Joules	Verapamil, 5 mg IV
↓	↓
Synchronous cardioversion 360 Joules	Verapamil, 10 mg IV
↓	(in 15-20 min)
Correct Underlying Abnormalities	↓
↓	Cardioversion, Digoxin,
Pharmacological Therapy + Cardioversion	β-Blockers, Pacing as Indicated

If conversion occurs but PSVT recurs, repeated electrical cardioversion is *not* indicated. Sedation should be used as time permits.

APPENDIX D

PEDIATRIC EMERGENCY DRUGS

SPECIAL CONSIDERATIONS: PEDIATRICS

The administration of life-saving medications to children presents several problems to emergency personnel. First, it is essential to estimate accurately the child's weight in kilograms. Most pediatric drug dosages are calculated based on the child's weight. Overestimation of body weight can lead to overdosage of the drug. Underestimation can cause less than therapeutic levels of the drug within the blood. Second, the drug dosages are often so small that dilution of the drug is often required. Finally, the physical size of the child sometimes makes administration difficult.

The pediatric drug dosages for the most commonly prescribed emergency drugs have been presented in Appendix A: Quick Drug Reference. The drugs in this section have been broken down and the dosage listed by specific patient weights. This will facilitate easy and rapid reference when confronted by a pediatric patient requiring pharmacological intervention.

HOW TO USE THIS SECTION

1. Estimate the patient's weight (often a fairly reliable weight can be obtained from the parents—or refer to Table D–1).
2. Convert the patient's weight to kilograms using Table D–2.

TABLE D–1   **Average Weight/Age for Pediatric Patients**

Age	Weight (lb)	Weight (kg)
Birth	7	3
3 mo	11	5
6 mo	15	7
9 mo	18	8
1 yr	22	10
2 yr	26	12
3 yr	33	15
4 yr	37	17
5 yr	40	18
6 yr	44	20
7 yr	50	23
8 yr	56	25
9 yr	60	28
10 yr	70	33
11 yr	75	35
12 yr	85	40
13 yr	98	44

TABLE D–2   **Conversion Table (Pounds = Kilograms)**

Pounds →	Kilograms	Pounds →	Kilograms	Pounds →	Kilograms
2.2	1	35.2	16	68.2	31
4.4	2	37.4	17	70.4	32
6.6	3	39.6	18	72.6	33
8.8	4	41.8	19	74.8	34
11	5	44	20	77	35
13.2	6	46.2	21	79.2	36
15.4	7	48.4	22	81.4	37
17.6	8	50.6	23	83.6	38
19.8	9	52.8	24	85.8	39
22	10	55	25	88	40
24.2	11	57.2	26	90.2	41
26.4	12	59.4	27	92.4	42
28.6	13	61.6	28	94.6	43
30.8	14	63.8	29	96.8	44
33	15	66	30	99	45

3. Consult the drug dosage chart beginning on page 266 and select the column that is closest to the patient's actual weight. The drug dosages for that weight are provided.

TABLE D-3 Drug Dosage Chart

	Body Weight (kg)				
	1	2	3	4	5
Atropine Sulfate	0.02 mg	0.04 mg	0.06 mg	0.08 mg	0.10 mg
Benadryl®	1.0 mg	2.0 mg	3.0 mg	4.0 mg	5.0 mg
Calcium Chloride	20.0 mg	40.0 mg	60.0 mg	80.0 mg	100.0 mg
Decadron®	0.3 mg	0.6 mg	0.9 mg	1.2 mg	1.5 mg
Dextrose 50%	0.5 g	1.0 g	1.5 g	2.0 g	2.5 g
Dopamine	5 µg/min	10 µg/min	15 µg/min	20 µg/min	25 µg/min
Epinephrine 1:10,000	0.01 mg	0.02 mg	0.03 mg	0.04 mg	0.05 mg
Isuprel®	0.1 µg/min	0.2 µg/min	0.3 µg/min	0.4 µg/min	0.5 µg/min
Lidocaine Bolus	1.0 mg	2.0 mg	3.0 mg	4.0 mg	5.0 mg
Lidocaine Infusion	30 µg/min	60 µg/min	90 µg/min	120 µg/min	150 µg/min
Narcan®	0.01 mg	0.02 mg	0.03 mg	0.04 mg	0.05 mg
Phenergan®	0.5 mg	1.0 mg	1.5 mg	2.0 mg	2.5 mg
Sodium Bicarbonate	1.0 mEq	2.0 mEq	3.0 mEq	4.0 mEq	5.0 mEq
Verapamil®	0.1 mg	0.2 mg	0.3 mg	0.4 mg	0.5 mg

6–10 Kg

TABLE D-3 Drug Dosage Chart (continued)

	Body Weight (kg)				
	6	7	8	9	10
Atropine Sulfate	0.12 mg	0.14 mg	0.16 mg	0.18 mg	0.20 mg
Benadryl®	6 mg	7 mg	8 mg	9 mg	10 mg
Calcium Chloride	120 mg	140 mg	160 mg	180 mg	200 mg
Decadron®	1.8 mg	2.1 mg	2.4 mg	2.7 mg	3.0 mg
Dextrose 50%	3.0 g	3.5 g	4.0 g	4.5 g	5.0 g
Dopamine	30 µg/min	35 µg/min	40 µg/min	45 µg/min	50 µg/min
Epinephrine 1:10,000	0.06 mg	0.07 mg	0.08 mg	0.09 mg	0.1 mg
Isuprel®	0.6 µg/min	0.7 µg/min	0.8 µg/min	0.9 µg/min	1 µg/min
Lidocaine Bolus	6 mg	7 mg	8 mg	9 mg	10 mg
Lidocaine Infusion	180 µg/min	210 µg/min	240 µg/min	270 µg/min	300 µg/min
Narcan®	0.06 mg	0.07 mg	0.08 mg	0.09 mg	0.10 mg
Phenergan®	3 mg	3.5 mg	4 mg	4.5 mg	5 mg
Sodium Bicarbonate	6 mEq	7 mEq	8 mEq	9 mEq	10 mEq
Verapamil®	0.6 mg	0.7 mg	0.8 mg	0.9 mg	1.0 mg

TABLE D-3   Drug Dosage Chart (continued)

11–15 Kg

	Body Weight (kg)				
	11	12	13	14	15
Atropine Sulfate	0.22 mg	0.24 mg	0.26 mg	0.28 mg	0.3 mg
Benadryl®	11 mg	12 mg	13 mg	14 mg	15 mg
Calcium Chloride	220 mg	240 mg	260 mg	280 mg	300 mg
Decadron®	3.3 mg	3.7 mg	4.0 mg	4.3 mg	4.6 mg
Dextrose 50%	5.5 g	6.0 g	6.5 g	7.0 g	7.5 g
Dopamine	55 µg/min	60 µg/min	65 µg/min	70 µg/min	75 µg/min
Epinephrine 1:10,000	0.11 mg	0.12 mg	0.13 mg	0.14 mg	0.15 mg
Isuprel®	1.1 µg/min	1.2 µg/min	1.3 µg/min	1.4 µg/min	1.5 µg/min
Lidocaine Bolus	11 mg	12 mg	13 mg	14 mg	15 mg
Lidocaine Infusion	330 µg/min	360 µg/min	390 µg/min	420 µg/min	450 µg/min
Narcan®	0.11 mg	0.12 mg	0.13 mg	0.14 mg	0.15 mg
Phenergan®	5.5 mg	6.0 mg	6.5 mg	7.0 mg	7.5 mg
Sodium Bicarbonate	11 mEq	12 mEq	13 mEq	14 mEq	15 mEq
Verapamil®	1.1 mg	1.2 mg	1.3 mg	1.4 mg	1.5 mg

TABLE D-3 Drug Dosage Chart (continued)

	Body Weight (kg)				
	16	17	18	19	20
Atropine Sulfate	0.32 mg	0.34 mg	0.36 mg	0.38 mg	0.4 mg
Benadryl®	16 mg	17 mg	18 mg	19 mg	20 mg
Calcium Chloride	320 mg	340 mg	360 mg	380 mg	400 mg
Decadron®	4.9 mg	5.0 mg	5.0 mg	5.0 mg	5.0 mg
Dextrose 50%	8.0 g	8.5 g	9.0 g	9.5 g	10 g
Dopamine	80 µg/min	85 µg/min	90 µg/min	95 µg/min	100 µg/min
Epinephrine 1:10,000	0.16 mg	0.17 mg	0.18 mg	0.19 mg	0.2 mg
Isuprel®	1.6 µg/min	1.7 µg/min	1.8 µg/min	1.9 µg/min	0.20 µg/min
Lidocaine Bolus	16 mg	17 mg	18 mg	19 mg	20 mg
Lidocaine Infusion	0.48 mg/min	0.51 mg/min	0.54 mg/min	0.57 mg/min	0.6 mg/min
Narcan®	0.16 mg	0.17 mg	0.18 mg	0.19 mg	0.2 mg
Phenergan®	8.0 mg	8.5 mg	9 mg	9.5 mg	10 mg
Sodium Bicarbonate	16 mEq	17 mEq	18 mEq	19 mEq	20 mEq
Verapamil®	1.6 mg	1.7 mg	1.8 mg	1.9 mg	2. mg

21–25 Kg

TABLE D-3 Drug Dosage Chart (continued)

	Body Weight (kg)				
	21	22	23	24	25
Atropine Sulfate	0.42 mg	0.44 mg	0.46 mg	0.48 mg	0.5 mg
Benadryl®	21 mg	22 mg	23 mg	24 mg	25 mg
Calcium Chloride	420 mg	440 mg	460 mg	480 mg	500 mg
Decadron®	5 mg	5 mg	5 mg	5 mg	5 mg
Dextrose 50%	10.5 g	11.0 g	11.5 g	12.0 g	12.5 g
Dopamine	105 µg/min	110 µg/min	115 µg/min	120 µg/min	125 µg/min
Epinephrine 1:10,000	0.21 mg	0.22 mg	0.23 mg	0.24 mg	0.25 mg
Isuprel®	2.1 µg/min	2.2 µg/min	2.3 µg/min	2.4 µg/min	2.5 µg/min
Lidocaine Bolus	21 mg	22 mg	23 mg	24 mg	25 mg
Lidocaine Infusion	0.63 mg/min	0.66 mg/min	0.69 mg/min	0.72 mg/min	0.75 mg/min
Narcan®	0.21 mg	0.22 mg	0.23 mg	0.24 mg	0.25 mg
Phenergan®	10.5 mg	11.0 mg	11.5 mg	12.0 mg	12.5 mg
Sodium Bicarbonate	21 mEq	22 mEq	23 mEq	24 mEq	25 mEq
Verapamil®	2.1 mg	2.2 mg	2.3 mg	2.4 mg	2.5 mg

TABLE D–3 Drug Dosage Chart (continued)

	Body Weight (kg)				
	26	27	28	29	30
Atropine Sulfate	0.5 mg	0.5 mg	0.5 mg	0.5 mg	0.5 mg
Benadryl®	26 mg	27 mg	28 mg	29 mg	30 mg
Calcium Chloride	500 mg	500 mg	500 mg	500 mg	500 mg
Decadron®	5 mg	5 mg	5 mg	5 mg	5 mg
Dextrose 50%	13.0 g	13.5 g	14.0 g	14.5 g	15.0 g
Dopamine	130 µg/min	135 µg/min	140 µg/min	145 µg/min	150 µg/min
Epinephrine 1:10,000	0.26 mg	0.27 mg	0.28 mg	0.29 mg	0.30 mg
Isuprel®	2.6 µg/min	2.7 µg/min	2.8 µg/min	2.9 µg/min	3.0 µg/min
Lidocaine Bolus	26 mg	27 mg	28 mg	29 mg	30 mg
Lidocaine Infusion	0.78 mg/min	0.81 mg/min	0.84 mg/min	0.87 mg/min	0.9 mg/min
Narcan®	0.26 mg	0.27 mg	0.28 mg	0.29 mg	0.30 mg
Phenergan®	13.0 mg	13.5 mg	14.0 mg	14.5 mg	15.0 mg
Sodium Bicarbonate	26 mEq	27 mEq	28 mEq	29 mEq	30 mEq
Verapamil®	2.6 mg	2.7 mg	2.8 mg	2.9 mg	3.0 mg

TABLE D-3   Drug Dosage Chart (continued)

	Body Weight (kg)				
	31	32	33	34	35
Atropine Sulfate	0.5 mg	0.5 mg	0.5 mg	0.5 mg	0.5 mg
Benadryl®	31 mg	32 mg	33 mg	34 mg	35 mg
Calcium Chloride	500 mg	500 mg	500 mg	500 mg	500 mg
Decadron®	5 mg	5 mg	5 mg	5 mg	5 mg
Dextrose 50%	15.5 g	16.0 g	16.5 g	17.0 g	17.5 g
Dopamine	155 µg/min	160 µg/min	165 µg/min	170 µg/min	175 µg/min
Epinephrine 1:10,000	0.31 mg	0.32 mg	0.33 mg	0.34 mg	0.35 mg
Isuprel®	3.1 µg/min	3.2 µg/min	3.3 µg/min	3.4 µg/min	3.5 µg/min
Lidocaine Bolus	31 mg	32 mg	33 mg	34 mg	35 mg
Lidocaine Infusion	0.93 mg/min	0.96 mg/min	0.99 mg/min	1.02 mg/min	1.05 mg/min
Narcan®	0.31 mg	0.32 mg	0.33 mg	0.34 mg	0.35 mg
Phenergan®	15.5 mg	16.0 mg	16.5 mg	17.0 mg	17.5 mg
Sodium Bicarbonate	31 mEq	32 mEq	33 mEq	34 mEq	35 mEq
Verapamil®	3.0 mg	3.0 mg	3.0 mg	3.0 mg	3.0 mg

36–40 Kg

TABLE D–3   Drug Dosage Chart (continued)

	Body Weight (kg)				
	36	37	38	39	40
Atropine Sulfate	0.5 mg	0.5 mg	0.5 mg	0.5 mg	0.5 mg
Benadryl®	36 mg	37 mg	38 mg	39 mg	40 mg
Calcium Chloride	500 mg	500 mg	500 mg	500 mg	500 mg
Decadron®	5 mg	5 mg	5 mg	5 mg	5 mg
Dextrose 50%	18.0 g	18.5 g	19.0 g	19.5 g	20.0 g
Dopamine	180 µg/min	185 µg/min	190 µg/min	195 µg/min	200 µg/min
Epinephrine 1:10,000	0.36 mg	0.37 mg	0.38 mg	0.39 mg	0.40 mg
Isuprel®	3.6 µg/min	3.7 µg/min	3.8 µg/min	3.9 µg/min	4.0 µg/min
Lidocaine Bolus	36 mg	37 mg	38 mg	39 mg	40 mg
Lidocaine Infusion	1.1 mg/min	1.1 mg/min	1.1 mg/min	1.2 mg/min	1.2 mg/min
Narcan®	0.36 mg	0.37 mg	0.38 mg	0.39 mg	0.4 mg
Phenergan®	18 mg	18.5 mg	19 mg	19.5 mg	20 mg
Sodium Bicarbonate	36 mEq	37 mEq	38 mEq	39 mEq	40 mEq
Verapamil®	3 mg	3 mg	3 mg	3 mg	3 mg

TABLE D–4   Resuscitation Medications, by Weight and Age, for Infants and Children 0–10 Years

Age	50th Percentile Weight (kg)	Epinephrine		Atropine		Bicarbonate[a]	
		mg	mL	mg	mL	mEq	mL
Newborn	3.0	0.03	0.3	0.1	1.0	3.0	6.0
1 Month	4.0	0.04	0.4	0.1	1.0	4.0	8.0
3 Months	5.5	0.055	0.55	0.11	1.1	5.5	11.0
6 Months	7.0	0.07	0.7	0.14	1.4	7.0	7.0
1 Year	10.0	0.10	1.0	0.20	2.0	10.0	10.0
2 Years	12.0	0.12	1.2	0.24	2.4	12.0	12.0
3 Years	14.0	0.14	1.4	0.28	2.8	14.0	14.0
4 Years	16.0	0.16	1.6	0.32	3.2	16.0	16.0
5 Years	18.0	0.18	1.8	0.36	3.6	18.0	18.0
6 Years	20.0	0.20	2.0	0.40	4.0	20.0	20.0
7 Years	22.0	0.22	2.2	0.44	4.4	22.0	22.0
8 Years	25.0	0.25	2.5	0.50	5.0	25.0	25.0
9 Years	28.0	0.28	2.8	0.56	5.6	28.0	28.0
10 Years	34.0	0.34	3.4	0.68	6.8	34.0	34.0

Volume (mL) is based on the following concentrations:

Epinephrine—1:10,000 (0.1 mg/mL)

Atropine—0.1 mg/mL

Bicarbonate—≤ 3 months = 4.2% solution (0.5 mEq/mL)

> 3 months = 8.4% solution (1 mEq/mL)

[a]The use of bicarbonate in cardiac arrest is controversial (see text). Good ventilation must be established before bicarbonate is used.

(Reproduced with permission. © Textbook of Pediatric Life Support, 1988, American Heart Association.)

**TABLE D–5   Infusion Medications, by Weight and Age, for Infants
and Children 0–10 Years**

ADD

0.6 mg (3 mL)[a] of **isoproterenol**
0.6 mg (0.6 mL)[a] of **epinephrine** | TO | 100 mL of diluent
60.0 mg (1.5 mL)[a] of **dopamine**
60.0 mg (2.4 mL)[a] of **dobutamine**

INFUSE

at 1 mL/kg/hr or according to following table in order

TO GIVE

0.1 μg/kg/min isoproterenol
0.1 μg/kg/min epinephrine
10 μg/kg/min dopamine
10 μg/kg/min dobutamine

Age	50th Percentile Weight (kg)	Infusion Rate (mL/hr)
Newborn	3	3
1 Month	4	4
3 Months	5.5	5.5
6 Months	7.0	7.0
1 Year	10.0	10.0
2 Years	12.0	12.0
3 Years	14.0	14.0
4 Years	16.0	16.0
5 Years	18.0	18.0
6 Years	20.0	20.0
7 Years	22.0	22.0
8 Years	25.0	25.0
9 Years	28.0	28.0
10 Years	34.0	34.0

These are starting doses. Adjust concentration to dose and fluid tolerance.

[a]Based on the following concentrations: isoproterenol = 0.2 mg/mL; epinephrine = 1:1000 (1 mg/mL); dopamine = 40 mg/mL; dobutamine = 25 mg/mL.

(Reproduced with permission. ©*Textbook of Pediatric Life Support*, 1988, American Heart Association.)

APPENDIX

HOME MEDICATION REFERENCE GUIDE

TABLE E–1 Home Medication Classes

Class	Actions
Analgesics	Raises pain threshold
	Alleviates anxiety and fear
	Alters physiological response to pain
Anorexiants	Controls appetite
Antacids	Reduce stomach and duodenal activity
	Raises stomach pH
Antianginals	Dilates peripheral and coronary arterioles
Antiarrhythmics	Suppresses ectopic activity
	Controls rhythm of heart
Antiarthritics	Controls joint inflammation and pain associated with arthritis
Antibiotics	Combats microorganisms
Anticoagulants	Prolongs blood-clotting time
Anticholinergics	Blocks actions of acetylcholine, thus potentiating sympathetic nervous system
Anticonvulsants	Suppresses seizure activity in the brain
	Suppresses spread of seizure activity in motor cortex
Antidepressants	Tricyclic compounds potentiate sympathetic effects by preventing the uptake of norepinephrine in the central nervous system
	Monoamine oxidase inhibitors prevent impulse transmission at the neurons and inhibit catecholamine breakdown
Antidiarrheal	Reduces bowel motility
Antiemetic	Relieves or prevents nausea and vomiting
	Stimulates H_2 histamine receptors
Antihistamines	Blocks release of histamine

TABLE E–1   Home Medication Classes (continued)

Class	Actions
Antihypertensives	Lowers blood pressure by sympathetic blockade
	Causes peripheral vasodilation
Antipsychotics	Phenothiazines are thought to block dopamine receptors in the brain associated with mood and behavior
Antispasmodics	Relieves pain
	Blocks acetylcholine in parts of the parasympathetic nervous system
Antituberculosis	Deactivates the tubercle bacillus
Bronchodilators	Relaxes smooth muscle of bronchioles
Cardiac Glycosides	Increases cardiac output
	Slows SA and AV conduction
	Positive inotrope
	Controls certain rhythm disorders
Diuretics	Stimulates release of water and sodium chloride from kidneys
	Inhibits reabsorption of sodium in nephron
Hypnotics	Induces sleep
and Sedatives	Depresses central nervous system
Hypoglycemics	Provides insulin to promote uptake of glucose by the cells
Laxatives and Stool	Stimulates peristalsis
Softeners	Alters fecal consistency
Steroids	Controls inflammatory response
Sulfamides	Antibiotics for urinary tract infections
Tranquilizers	Induces calmness without depression of level of consciousness
	Depresses central nervous system

TABLE E–2   Common Home Medications[a]

Medication	Use
A/T/S	Topical antibiotic
Accutane	Acne agent
acetaminophen	Analgesic
acetazolamide	Diuretic
Achromycin	Antibiotic
Actibine	Impotence agent
Actifed	Antihistamine and decongestant
Acyclovir	Antiviral
Adalat	Calcium channel blocker
Adipex	Appetite suppressant
Aerobid	Steroid inhaler
Agyestin	Progesterone
Akineton	Anti-Parkinson agent
albuterol	Bronchodilator
Aldactazide	Diuretic
Aldactone	Diuretic
Aldoclor	Antihypertensive and diuretic
Aldomet	Antihypertensive
Aldoril	Antihypertensive and diuretic

TABLE E–2   **Common Home Medications**[a] **(continued)**

Medication	Use
allopurinol	Antigout
alprazolam	Benzodiazepine
Alupent	Bronchodilator
amantadine	Antiparkinson agent and antiviral
Ambenyl	Narcotic cough suppressant
Amen	Progesterone
amiloride	Diuretic
Aminophyllin	Theophylline
amitriptyline	Tricyclic antidepressant
amoxapine	Antidepressant
amoxicillin	Antibiotic
Amoxil	Antibiotic
Anaprox	Analgesic and antiarthritic
Anexia	Analgesic
Ansaid	Antiarthritic
Anspor	Antibiotic
Antabuse	Antialcoholism agent
Anturane	Antigout
Apresazide	Antihypertensive and diuretic
Apresoline	Antihypertensive
Aristocort	Steroid
Artane	Anti-Parkinson
Asendin	Antidepressant
aspirin	Analgesic
astemizole	Antihistamine
Astramorph	Narcotic
Atarax	Antihistamine
atenolol	β Blocker
Ativan	Benzodiazepine
Atrohist	Antihistamine
Atromid	Lipid-lowering agent
Atrovent	Bronchodilator
Augmentin	Antibiotic
Axid	Antiulcer
Axotal	Analgesic
azathioprine	Immunosuppressant
Azdone	Narcotic analgesic
Bactrim	Antibiotic
Bactroban	Antibiotic
Bancap HC	Narcotic analgesic
beclomethasone	Steroid
Beclovent	Steroid inhaler
Beconase	Steroid
Benadryl	Antihistamine
Benemid	Antigout
Bentyl	Gastrointestinal antispasmodic
benzonatate	Cough suppressant
benzotropine	Anti-Parkinson
Betaoptic	Antiglaucoma and β blocker

TABLE E–2   **Common Home Medications^a (continued)**

Medication	Use
betaxolol	Antiglaucoma and β blocker
Bicillin	Antibiotic
Blocadren	β Blocker
Bontril	Appetite suppressant
Breathaire	Bronchodilator
Brethine	Bronchodilator
Brevicon	Birth control
Bricanyl	Bronchodilator
bromocriptine	Anti-Parkinson
brompheniramine	Antihistamine
Bronkodyl	Theophylline
Buprenex	Narcotic analgesic
bupropion	Antidepressant
Buspar	Anxiolytic
buspirone	Anxiolytic
butalbital	Analgesic
Butazolidin	Antiarthritic
Butisol	Hypnotic
Cafergot	Migraine headache agent
Calan	Calcium channel blocker
Cantil	Antiulcer
Capital	analgesic
Capoten	Antihypertensive
Capozide	Antihypertensive and diuretic
captopril	Antihypertensive
Carafate	Antiulcer
carbamazepine	Anticonvulsant
carbidopa	Anti-Parkinson
Cardene	Calcium channel blocker
Cardilate	Antianginal
Cardizem	Calcium channel blocker
carisoprodol	Muscle relaxant
carteolol	β Blocker
Cartrol	β Blocker
Catapres	Antihypertensive
Ceclor	Antibiotic
Cedilanid	Digitalis
cefaclor	Antibiotic
cefadroxil	Antibiotic
cefixime	Antibiotic
Ceftin	Antibiotic
cefuroxime	Antibiotic
Centrax	Benzodiazepine
Cesamet	Antiemetic
chlordiazepoxide	Benzodiazepine
Chloromycetin	Antibiotic
chlorpromazine	Antiulcer
chlorpropamide	Oral hypoglycemic agent
chlorthalidone	Diuretic

TABLE E–2   Common Home Medications^a (continued)

Medication	Use
Choledyl	Theophylline
cholestyramine	Lipid lowering agent
Choloxin	Thyroid preparation
Chronulac	Laxative
Cibalith	Lithium (antimania)
cimetadine	Antiulcer
Cinobac	Antibiotic
Cipro	Antibiotic
ciprofloxacin	Antibiotic
Cleocin	Antibiotic
clindamycin	Antibiotic
Clinoril	Antiarthritic
clofazimine	Antileprosy
clofibrate	Lipid lowering agent
clonazepam	Antiseizure and benzodiazepine
clonidine	Antihypertensive
clorazepate	Benzodiazepine
Codiclear	Narcotic cough suppressant
Codimal	Decongestant
Cogentin	Anti-Parkinson
ColBENEMID	Antigout
Colace	Stool softener
Combipress	Antihypertensive and diuretic
Comhist	Antihistamine and decongestant
Comtrex	Decongestant
Constant-T	Theophylline
Cordarone	Antiarrhythmic
Corgard	β Blocker
Corzide	β Blocker/diuretic
Coumadin	Anticoagulant
cromolyn sodium	Allergy suppressant
Crystodigin	Digitalis
Cyclert	Central nervous system stimulant
cyclizine	Antiemetic
cycloserine	Antituberculosis
cycobenzaprine	Muscle relaxant
Cycrin	Progesterone
cyproheptadine	Antihistamine
Cystospaz	Urinary antispasmodic
Cytadren	Adrenal suppressant
Cytomel	Thyroid
Cytotec	Antiulcer
Dalmane	Benzodiazepine
Damason	Analgesic
Dantrium	Antispasmodic
Dapsone	Antileprosy
Daraprim	Antiparasitic
Darbid	Antiulcer
Darvon	Narcotic-type analgesic

TABLE E–2   **Common Home Medications**[a] **(continued)**

Medication	Use
Datril	Antiarthritic
Decadron	Steroid
Declomycin	Antibiotic
Deconamine	Decongestant
Deconsal	Decongestant
Delsym	Cough suppressant
Deltasone	Steroid
democycline	Antibiotic
Demulen	Birth control
Depakene	Anticonvulsant
Depakote	Anticonvulsant
Deponit	Nitroglycerin antianginal
deserpidine	Antihypertensive
desipramine	Tricyclic antidepressant
Desoxyn	Amphetamine
Desyrel	Antidepressant
dexamethasone	Steroid
Dexedrine	Amphetamine
Diabeta	Oral hypoglycemic
Diabinase	Oral hypoglycemic agent
Diamox	Diuretic
diazepam	Benzodiazepine
diclofenac	Antiarthritic
Dicumarol	Anticoagulant
dicyclomine	Gastrointestinal antispasmodic
Didrex	Appetite suppressant
diethylproprion	Appetite suppressant
diethylstilbestrol	Estrogen
diflunisal	Antiarthritic
digoxin	Digitalis
Dilantin	Anticonvulsant
Dilatrate	Antianginal
Dilaudid	Narcotic analgesic
Dilor	Theophylline
diltiazem	Calcium channel blocker
Dimetame	Decongestant
diphenhydramine	Antihistamine
dipyridamone	Anticoagulant
Disalcid	Antiarthritic
disopyramide	Antiarrhythmic
disopyramide	Antiarrhythmic
disulfirim	Antialcoholism agent
Ditropan	Bladder antispasmodic
Diulo	Diuretic
Diupres	Antihypertensive and diuretic
Diurel	Diuretic
Diutensin	Antihypertensive
divalproex sodium	Anticonvulsant
docusate	Laxative

TABLE E–2   Common Home Medications[a] **(continued)**

Medication	Use
Dolobid	Antiarthritic
Dolophine	Narcotic
Donnatal	Gastrointestinal antispasmodic
Doral	Benzodiazepine
Doriden	Hypnotic
Dorx	Antibiotic
doxepin	Antidepressant
doxycycline	Antibiotic
Dramamine	Antihistamine
Dulcolax	Laxative
Duocet	Analgesic
Dura-Vent	Decongestant
Duricef	Antibiotic
Dyazide	Diuretic
Dyrenium	Diuretic
E.E.S.	Antibiotic
Easprin	Aspirin
Ecotrin	Aspirin
Edecrin	Diuretic
Elavil	Tricyclic antidepressant
Eldepryl	Anti-Parkinson agent
Elixophyllin	Theophylline
Emetrol	Antiemetic
Empirin	Analgesic
encainaide	Antiarrhythmic
Endep	Tricyclic antidepressant
Enduron	Diuretic
Enduronyl	Antihypertensive and diuretic
Enkaid	Antiarrhythmic
Enovid	Birth control
Entex	Decongestant
Entolase	Digestive enzyme supplement
Ergostat	Migraine headache agent
ERYC	Antibiotic
Eryderm	Topical antibiotic
erythrityl	Antianginal
Erythrocin	Antibiotic
erythromycin	Antibiotic
Ery-Tab	Antibiotic
Esgic	Analgesic
Esidrix	Diuretic
Eskalith	Antimania agent
Esmil	Antihypertensive and diuretic
Estinyl	Estrogen
Estrace	Estrogen
Estraderm	Estrogen
estradiol	Estrogen
Estratab	Estrogen
estropipate	Estrogen

TABLE E-2   Common Home Medications[a] (continued)

Medication	Use
Estrovis	Estrogen
ethacrynic acid	Diuretic
Ethatab	Vasodilator
ethaverine	Vasodilator
ethchlorvynol	Hypnotic
ethinamate	Hypnotic
Ethmozine	Antiarrhythmic
ethosuximide	Antiseizure
ethotoin	Anticonvulsant
Etrafon	Antianxiety and tricyclic antidepressant
Euthroid	Thyroid
E-mycin	Antibiotic
famotidine	Antiulcer
Fastin	Appetite suppressant
Feldene	Antiarthritic
fenfluramine	Appetite suppressant
Feosol	Iron
Fergon	Iron
Fero-Folic	Iron tablets
Fero-Grad	Iron tablets
Fero-Gradumer	Iron tablets
Fioricet	Analgesic
Fiorinal	Analgesic
Flagyl	Antibiotic
flecanine	Antiarrhythmic
Flexeril	Muscle relaxant
fluoxetine	Antidepressant
fluphenazine	Antipsychotic
flurazepam	Benzodiazepine
flurbiprofen	Antiarthritic
Fulvicin	Antifungal
furazolidone	Antibiotic
furosemide	Diuretic
Furoxone	Antibiotic
Gantrisin	Antibiotic
gemfibrozil	Lipid-lowering agent
Genora	Birth control
Geocillin	Antibiotic
glipizide	Oral hypoglycemic agent
Glucotrol	Oral hypoglycemic agent
glyburide	Oral hypoglycemic
glycopyrrolate	Antiulcer
Grisactin	Antifungal
guanethidine	Antihypertensive
guanfacine	Antihypertensive
Halcion	Benzodiazepine
Haldol	Antipsychotic
haloperidol	Antipsychotic
Harmonyl	Antihypertensive

TABLE E–2   **Common Home Medications**^a **(continued)**

Medication	Use
Hexadrol	Steroid
Hismanal	Antihistamine
Histaspan	Antihistamine
Humibid	Decongestant
Humulin R	Insulin
Humulin N	Insulin
Hycodan	Narcotic cough suppressant
hycomine	Narcotic cough suppressant
Hycotuss	Narcotic cough suppressant
hydralazine	Antihypertensive
Hydrocet	Narcotic analgesic
hydrochlorthiazide	Diuretic
hydrocodone	Analgesic
Hydrocortone	Steroid
HydroDIURIL	Diuretic
hydroflumethazide	Diuretic
hydromorphone	Narcotic analgesic
Hydromox	Diuretic
Hydromox	Antihypertensive and diuretic
Hydropres	Antihypertensive and diuretic
hydroxyzine	Antihistamine
Hygroton	Diuretic
Hytrin	Antihypertensive
Iberet-Folic-500	Iron tablets
ibuprofen	Antiarthritic
Ilosone	Antibiotic
Ilotycin	Antibiotic
imipramine	Tricyclic antidepressant
Imodium	Antidiarrheal
Imodium A-D	Antidiarrheal
Imuran	Immunosuppressant
indapamide	Antihypertensive
Inderal	β Blocker
Inderide	β Blocker and diuretic
Indocin	Antiarthritic
indomethacin	Antiarthritic
INH	Antituberculosis
Insulatard	Insulin
Intal	Allergy suppressant
Inversine	Antihypertensive
ipratropium	Bronchodilator
Ismelin	Antihypertensive
isocarboxazid	Antidepressant (monoamine oxidase inhibitor)
isoproterenol	Bronchodilator
Isoptin	Calcium channel blocker
isorbide	Antianginal
Isordil	Antianginal
isotretinoin	Acne agent

TABLE E–2   **Common Home Medications**[a] **(continued)**

Medication	Use
Janimine	Tricyclic antidepressant
Kaochlor	Potassium supplement
Kaon	Potassium supplement
Kaopectate	Antidiarrheal
Kato	Potassium supplement
Keflit	Antibiotic
Keftab	Antibiotic
Kemadrin	Anti-Parkinson agent
ketoconazole	Antifungal
ketoprofen	Antiarthritic
Kinesed	Antiulcer
Klonapin	Antiseizure/Benzodiazepine
Klorvess	Potassium supplement
Klor-Con	Potassium supplement
Klotrix	Potassium supplement
K-DUR	Potassium supplement
K-Lor	Potassium supplement
K-Lyte	Potassium supplement
K-Phos	Urinary acidifier
K-Tab	Potassium supplement
labetalol	β Blocker
Lamprene	Antileprosy
Lanoxicaps	Digitalis
Lanoxin	Digitalis
Larodopa	Anti-Parkinson
Lasix	Diuretic
Lente	Insulin
Levatol	β Blocker
levodopa	Anti-Parkinson
Levothroid	Thyroid
Levoxine	Thyroid
Librax	Gastrointestinal antispasmodic/Benzodiazepine
Librium	Benzodiazepine
lidocaine	Local anesthetic
Lincocin	Antibiotic
lincomycin	Antibiotic
Lioresal	Muscle relaxant
lisinopril	Antihypertensive
Lithane	Antimania agent
Lithobid	Lithium (antimania)
Lo/Ovral	Birth control
Loestrin	Birth control
Lomotil	Antidiarrheal
Loniten	Antihypertensive
loperamide	Antidiarrheal
Lopid	Lipid-lowering agent
Lopressor	β Blocker
lorazepam	Benzodiazepine

TABLE E–2 **Common Home Medications**[a] **(continued)**

Medication	Use
Lorelco	Cholesterol-lowering agent
Lortab	Narcotic analgesic
lovastatin	Cholesterol-lowering agent
loxapine	Antipsychotic
Loxitane	Antipsychotic
Lozol	Antihypertensive
Ludiomil	Antidepressant
Lufyllin	Theophylline
Macrodantin	Antibiotic
Magan	Antiarthritic
magnesium salicylate	Antiarthritic
maprotiline	Antidepressant
Marax	Bronchodilator
Marezine	Antiemetic
Marinol	Antiemetic
Marplan	Antidepressant (monoamine oxidase inhibitor)
Materna	Vitamins
Maxair	Inhaled bronchodilator
Maxzide	Diuretic
Mebaral	Barbiturate hypnotic
mebendazole	Antiparasitic
mecamylamine	Antihypertensive
meclofenamate	Antiarthritic
Meclomen	Antiarthritic
Medrol	Steroid
mefenmic	Analgesic
Mellaril	Antipsychotic
mepenzolate	Antiulcer
meprobamate	Anxiolytic
Mesantoin	Anticonvulsant
mesoridazine	Antipsychotic
Mestinon	Myasthenia gravis agent
Metandren	Testosterone
Metaprel	Bronchodilator
metaproterenol	Bronchodilator
methadone	Narcotic
methamphetamine	Amphetamine
methocarbamol	Muscle relaxant
Methotrexate	Antiarthritic
methyclothiazide	Diuretic
methyldopa	Antihypertensive
methylphenidate	Central nervous system stimulant
metoclopramide	Gastric stimulant
metolazone	Antihypertensive
metoprolol	β Blocker
metronidazole	Antibiotic
Mevacor	Cholesterol-lowering agent
mexiletine	Antiarrhythmic

TABLE E–2   **Common Home Medications**[a] **(continued)**

Medication	Use
Mexitil	Antiarrhythmic
Micro K	Potassium supplement
Micronase	Oral antihypoglycemic agent
Micronor	Birth control
Midamor	Diuretic
Midrin	Analgesic
Milontin	Antiseizure
Miltown	Anxiolytic
Minipress	Antihypertensive
Minitran	Nitroglycerin antianginal
Minizide	Antihypertensive and diuretic
Minocin	Antibiotic
minocycline	Antibiotic
minoxidil	Antihypertensive
misprostol	Antiulcer
Mixtard	Insulin
Moban	Antipsychotic
Modane	Laxative
Moderil	Antihypertensive
Modicon	Birth control
Moduretic	Diuretic
molindone	Antipsychotic
Mongesic	Antiarthritic
moricizine	Antiarrhythmic
Motofen	Antidiarrheal
Motrin	Antiarthritic
MS Contin	Narcotic analgesic
MSIR	Narcotic analgesic
Myambutol	Antituberculosis
Mycostatin	Antifungal
Mykrox	Antihypertensive
Mysoline	Antiseizure
nabilone	Antiemetic
nadolol	β Blocker
Naldecon	Decongestant
Nalfon	Antiarthritic
Naphcon	Opthalmic antihistamine and decongestant
Naprosyn	Antiarthritic
Nardil	Antidepressant (monoamine oxidase inhibitor)
Nasalcrom	Allergy suppressant
Nasalide	Steroid
Natalins	Vitamins
Naturetin	Diuretic
Navane	Antipsychotic
Nembutal	Barbiturate
Neosporin	Topical antibiotic
nicardipine	Calcium channel blocker
Niclocide	Antiparasitic

TABLE E–2   **Common Home Medications**[a] **(continued)**

Medication	Use
Nicorette	Nicotine gum
nifedipine	Calcium channel blocker
nimodipine	Calcium channel blocker
Nimotop	Calcium channel blocker
Nitrgard	Nitroglycerin antianginal
Nitrodisc	Nitroglycerin antianginal
nitrofurantoin	Antibiotic
nitroglycerin	Antianginal
Nitrol	Nitroglycerin antianginal
Nitrolingual	Nitroglycerin antianginal
Nitrospan	Nitroglycerin antianginal
Nitrostat	Nitroglycerin antianginal
Nitro-Bid	Nitroglycerin antianginal
Nitro-Dur	Nitroglycerin antianginal
Nix	Antiparasitic (lice)
nizatidine	Antiulcer
Nizoral	Antifungal
Nolamine	Decongestant
Nolex	Decongestant
Noluldar	Hypnotic
Norcept	Birth control
Nordette–21	Birth control
Norethin	Birth control
Norflex	Muscle relaxant
Norgesic	Analgesic
Norinyl	Birth control
Norisodrine	Bronchodilator
Norlestrin	Birth control
Norlutate	Progesterone
Norlutin	Progesterone
Normodyne	β blocker
Normozide	β blocker and diuretic
norfloxacin	Antibiotic
Noroxin	Antibiotic
Norpace	Antiarrhythmic
Norpramin	Tricyclic antidepressant
nortriptyline	Tricyclic antidepressant
Norzine	Antiemetic
Novafed	Decongestant
Novahistine	Decongestant and antihistamine
Novolin	Insulin
Nucofed	Narcotic cough suppressant
Octamide	Gastric stimulant
Ogen	Estrogen
Omnipen	Antibiotic
Orap	Antipsychotic
Oretic	Diuretic
Oreticyl	Antihypertensive and diuretic
Organidin	Decongestant

TABLE E–2 Common Home Medications[a] **(continued)**

Medication	Use
Orinase	Oral hypoglycemic agent
Ornade	Decongestant and antihistamine
orphrnadrine	Muscle relaxant
Ortho-Novum	Birth control
Orudis	Antiarthritic
Ovcon	Birth control
Ovral	Estrogen
Ovral–28	Birth control
oxazepam	Benzodiazepine
oxybutynin	Bladder antispasmodic
oxycodone	Narcotic analgesic
oxytetracycline	Antibiotic
Pamelor	Tricyclic antidepressant
Pancrease	Digestive enzyme supplement
pancrelipase	Digestive enzyme supplement
Panwarfin	Anticoagulant
Paradione	Antiseizure
Parafon Forte	Muscle relaxant
paramethadione	Antiseizure
Parlodel	Anti-Parkinson
Parnate	Antidepressant (monoamine oxidase inhibitor)
Pavabid	Peripheral vascular antispasmodic
PBZ	Antihistamine
PCE	Antibiotic
Pediacare	Decongestant and antihistamine
Pediapred	Steroid
Pediazole	Antibiotic
Peganone	Anticonvulsant
pemoline	Central nervous system stimulant
penicillin	Antibiotic
Penntuss	Narcotic cough suppressant
pentazocine	Narcotic-like analgesic
Pentids	Antibiotic
pentobarbital	Barbiturate
pentoxifylline	Decreases blood viscosity
Pepcid	Antiulcer
Percocet	Narcotic analgesic
Percodan	Narcotic analgesic
Periactin	Antihistamine
Peritrate	Antianginal
Peri-Colace	Stool softener and laxative
Permax	Anti-Parkinson
Permitil	Antipsychotic
Persantine	Anticoagulant
Pertofrane	Antidepressant
Pfizerpen	Antibiotic
phenacemide	Anticonvulsant
Phenaphen	Analgesic

TABLE E–2   **Common Home Medications**[a] **(continued)**

Medication	Use
phenazopyridine	Urinary tract analgesic
phenelzine	Antidepressant (monoamine oxidase inhibitor)
Phenergan	Antiemetic
phenmetrazine	Appetite suppressant
phenolphthalein	Laxative
phensuximide	Antiseizure
phentermine	Appetite suppressant
Phenurone	Anticonvulsant
phenylbutazone	Antiarthritic
phenyltoloxoamine	Antihistamine
phenytoin	Anticonvulsant
pheytoin	Anticonvulsant
pimozide	Antipsychotic
pindolol	β Blocker
piroxicam	Antiarthritic
Placidyl	Hypnotic
Plegine	Appetite suppressant
PMB	Estrogen
Polaramine	Antihistamine
Polysporin	Topical antibiotic
Pondimin	Appetite suppressant
Ponstel	Analgesic
potassium chloride	Potassium supplement
prazepam	Benzodiazepine
prazosin	Antihypertensive
prednisolone	Steroid
prednisone	Steroid
Preluden	Appetite suppressant
Premarin	Estrogen
Primatene	Inhaled bronchodilator
primidone	Antiseizure
Principen	Antibiotic
Prinivil	Antihypertensive
Prinzide	Antihypertensive and diuretic
probenecid	Antigout
probucol	Cholesterol-lowering agent
procainamide	Antiarrhythmic
Procan SR	Antiarrhythmic
Procardia	Antihypertensive and antianginal
procyclidine	Anti-Parkinson agent
Prolixin	Antipsychotic
Proloid	Thyroid
promethazine	Antiemetic
Pronestyl	Antiarrhythmic
propafenone	Antiarrhythmic
Propagest	Decongestant
propoxyphene	Narcotic-type analgesic
propranolol	β Blocker

TABLE E–2   Common Home Medications^a (continued)

Medication	Use
Protostat	Antibiotic
protriptyline	Antidepressant
Proventil	Bronchodilator
Provera	Progesterone
Prozac	Antidepressant
Pro-Banthine	Antiulcer
pseudoephedrine	Decongestant
PV Tussin	Narcotic cough suppressant
Pyridium	Urinary tract analgesic
pyridostigmine	Myasthenia gravis agent
Quadrinal	Combination bronchodilator
Quarzan	Antiulcer
quazepam	Benzodiazepine
Questran	Lipid-lowering agent
Quibron	Theophylline
Quinamm	Muscle cramp analgesic
quinethazone	Diuretic
Quinidex	Antiarrhythmic
quinidine	Antiarrhythmic
Quiniglute	Antiarrhythmic
Quinora	Antiarrhythmic
ranitidine	Antiulcer
Raudixin	Antihypertensive
Rauzide	Antihypertensive and diuretic
Regitine	Antihypertensive
Reglan	Stomach stimulant
Regroton	Antihypertensive
Renese	Antihypertensive and diuretic
reserpine	Antihypertensive
Respid	Theophylline
Restoril	Benzodiazepine
Retrovir	Antiviral agent (AIDS)
Ridaura	Antiarthritic (gold)
Rifadin	Antituberculosis
Rifamate	Antituberculosis
Rimactane	Antibiotic
Ritalin	Central nervous system stimulant
ritodrine	Tocolytic (suppresses labor)
Robaxin	Muscle relaxant
Robinul	Antiulcer
Rogaine	Baldness treatment
Rondec	Decongestant
Roxanol	Narcotic analgesic
Rufen	Antiarthritic
Ru-Tuss	Cough and decongestant
Rynatuss	Cough suppressant and decongestant
Rythmol	Antiarrhythmic
Salflex	Antiarthritic

TABLE E–2   Common Home Medications*a* (continued)

Medication	Use
salsalate	Antiarthritic
Saluron	Diuretic
Salutensin	Antihypertensive and diuretic
Sanorex	Appetite suppressant
Seldane	Antihistamine
Semilente	Insulin
Septra	Antibiotic
Serax	Benzodiazepine
Serentil	Antipsychotic
Seromycin	Antituberculosis
Serpasil	Antihypertensive
SER-AP-ES	Antihypertensive
Sinemet	Anti-Parkinson
Sinequan	Antidepressant
Sinulin	Decongestant
Skelaxin	Muscle relaxant
Slo-Bid	Theophylline
Slo-Phyllin	Theophylline
Soma	Muscle relaxant
Spectrobid	Antibiotic
spironolactone	Diuretic
Stelazine	Antipsychotic
sucralfate	Antiulcer
Sudafed	Decongestant
sulfamethoxazole	Antibiotic
sulfinpyrazone	Antigout
sulfisoxazole	Antibiotic
sulindac	Antiarthritic
Sumycin	Antibiotic
Suprax	Antibiotic
Surbex	Vitamin
Surmontil	Tricyclic antidepressant
Symmetrel	Anti-Parkinson and antiviral
Synalgos-DC	Narcotic analgesic
Synthroid	Thyroid preparation
Tagamet	Antiulcer
Talwin	Narcotic-like analgesic
Tambocor	Antiarrhythmic
TAO	Antibiotic
Tavist	Antihistamine
Tegretol	Anticonvulsant
temazepam	Benzodiazepine
Tenex	Antihypertensive
Tenoretic	β Blocker and diuretic
Tenormin	β Blocker
Tenuate	Appetite suppressant
Ten-K	Potassium supplement
Tepanil	Appetite suppressant
terazosin	Antihypertensive

TABLE E–2   Common Home Medications^a (continued)

Medication	Use
terbutaline	Bronchodilator
terfenadine	Antihistamine
Terramycin	Antibiotic
Tessalon	Cough suppressant
tetracycline	Antibiotic
Thalitone	Diuretic
Theobid	Theophylline bronchodilator
Theochron	Theophylline
Theoclear	Theophylline
Theolair	Theophylline
Theo-24	Theophylline
Theo-Dur	Theophylline
thiordazine	Antipsychotic
thiothixene	Antipsychotic
Thorazine	Antiulcer
Tigan	Antiemetic
Timolide	β Blocker and antihypertensive
timolol	β Blocker
tocainaide	Antiarrhythmic
Tofranil	Tricyclic antidepressant
tolazamide	Oral hypoglycemic agent
tolbutamide	Oral hypoglycemic agent
Tolectin	Antiarthritic
Tolinase	Oral hypoglycemic agent
Toncard	Antiarrhythmic
Toradol	Analgesic
Torecan	Antiemetic
Tornalate	Inhaled bronchodilator
Trancopal	Anxiolytic
Trandate	β Blocker
Transderm-Nitro	Nitroglycerin antianginal
Transdern SCOP	Antiemetic
Tranxene	Benzodiazepine
tranylcypromine	Antidepressant (monoamine oxidase inhibitor)
trazadone	Antidepressant
Trecator	Antituberculosis
Trental	Decreases blood viscosity
triamcinolone	Steroid
Triaminic	Decongestant
triamterene	Diuretic
Triavil	Tricyclic antidepressant
triazolam	Benzodiazepine
Tridil	Nitroglycerin antianginal
Tridione	Anticonvulsant
trifluoperazine	Antipsychotic
trihexyphenidyl	Anti-Parkinson
Trilafon	Antipsychotic
Trilisate	Antiarthritic

TABLE E–2   Common Home Medications^a (continued)

Medication	Use
trimethadione	Anticonvulsant
trimethobenzamide	Antiemetic
Trimox	Antibiotic
Trimpex	Antibiotic
trimpramine	Tricyclic antidepressant
trimrthoprim	Antibiotic
Trinalin	Antihistamine
Triphasil	Birth control
Tri-Levlen	Birth control
Tri-norinyl	Birth control
Tussigon	Narcotic cough suppressant
Tussionex	Narcotic cough suppressant
Tussi-Organidin	Cough suppressant
Tylenol with Codeine	Narcotic analgesic
Tylenol	Analgesic
Tylox	Narcotic analgesic
Tympagesic	Ear anesthetic
Ultracef	Antibiotic
Unipen	Antibiotic
Uniphyl	Theophylline
Urecholine	Bladder antispasmodic
Urised	Urinary antispasmodic
Urispas	Urinary antispasmodic
Valium	Benzodiazepine
Valmid	Hypnotic
Valpin	Antiulcer
valproic acid	Anticonvulsant
Valrelease	Benzodiazepine
Vancenase	Steroid
Vanceril	Steroid
Vanocin	Antibiotic
vancomycin	Antibiotic
Vasoretic	Antihypertensive and diuretic
Vasotec	Antihypertensive
Veetids	Antibiotic
Velosef	Antibiotic
Velosulin	Insulin
Ventolin	Bronchodilator
verapamil	Calcium channel blocker
Verelan	Calcium channel blocker
Vermox	Antiparasitic
Vibramycin	Antibiotic
Vicodin	Narcotic analgesic
Vicon	Vitamin
Visken	β Blocker
Vistaril	Antihistamine
Vivactil	Antidepressant
Voltaren	Antiarthritic
Vontrol	Antiemetic

TABLE E–2   Common Home Medications^a (continued)

Medication	Use
warfarin	Anticoagulant
Wellbutrin	Antidepressant
Wigraine	Migraine headache agent
Wycillin	Antibiotic
Wygesic	Analgesic
Wymox	Antibiotic
Wymycin	Antibiotic
Wytensin	Antihypertensive
Xanax	Benzodiazepine
Xylocaine	Local anesthetic
yohimbine	Impotence agent
Yohimex	Impotence agent
Yutopar	Tocolytic (suppresses labor)
Zantac	Antiulcer
Zarontin	Antiseizure
Zestoretic	Antihypertensive and diuretic
Zestril	Antihypertensive
zidovudine	Antiviral agent (AIDS)
ZORprin	Aspirin
Zovirax	Antiviral
Zydone	Narcotic analgesic
Zyloprim	Antigout
Zymase	Digestive enzyme supplement

^{a}Listing of the most commonly prescribed medications. If additional information is required concerning a drug, consult the *Physician's Desk Reference* or a similar source. Trade names are capitalized, and generic names are lowercased.

APPENDIX F

ADDITIONAL PRACTICE PROBLEMS

PRACTICE CONVERSIONS

Convert the following:

1. 750 grams = _____ kilogram
2. ¾ grain = _____ milligrams
3. 0.65 liter = _____ milliliters
4. 100 micrograms = _____ milligram
5. 168 pounds = _____ kilograms
6. 43 inches = _____ centimeters
7. 2.75 liters = _____ milliliters
8. 68°F = _____ °C
9. 1¼ grain = _____ milligrams
10. 375 cubic centimeters = _____ milliliters
11. 18 pounds = _____ kilograms
12. 1 kiloliter = _____ liters
13. 45°C = _____ °F
14. 15 milligrams = _____ grains
15. 300 milligrams = _____ grains

DRUG DOSAGE CALCULATIONS

Calculate the following:

1. You are to administer 25 milligrams of lidocaine by IV bolus to a patient. Lidocaine is supplied in prefilled syringes containing 100 milligrams in 5 milliliters. How many milliliters do you administer?

2. You are ordered to administer 20 milligrams of labetalol to a patient by IV bolus. Labetalol is supplied in ampules containing 100 milligrams of the drug in 20 milliliters of solvent. How many milliliters of the drug do you administer?

3. The base-station physician wants you to administer 2 milligrams of morphine intravenously to an elderly patient after you have made a 10:1 dilution with D_5W solution. Your ampule contains 10 milligrams of morphine in 1 milliliter of solvent. How many milliliters do you administer?

4. A physician wants you to administer a quarter of grain of morphine to a patient. The ampule contains 10 milligrams of the drug in 1 milliliter of solvent. How many milliliters of the drug do you administer?

5. You are to prepare an infusion of labetalol. You are asked to put two ampules of labetalol in 250 milliliters of D_5W. Labetalol is supplied in ampules containing 100 milligrams in 20 milliliters of solvent. After you prepare the infusion, what will be the concentration of the infusion?

6. Using the solution prepared in problem 5, how many drops per minute do you infuse to deliver 2 milligrams per minute using a minidrip administration set?

7. You are to administer 1 liter of 0.9% sodium chloride solution to a patient over a 2-hour period. Using a standard administration set, how many drops per minute do you infuse?

8. You are to administer 0.75 milligram of bumetanide by IV bolus to a patient. The drug is supplied in vials containing 0.5 milligrams of the drug in 2 milliliters of solvent. How many milliliters of the drug do you administer?

9. A 244-pound patient is suffering a hypertensive crisis. The base-station physician wants you to administer a sodium nitroprusside infusion to the patient at a dose of 3 micrograms per kilogram per minute. If you place 50 milligrams of the drug in 500 milliliters of D_5W, how many drops per minute will you administer using a minidrip set?

10. A physician wants you to administer 0.75 milligrams per kilogram of amrinone by IV bolus to a patient in severe congestive heart failure. Amrinone is supplied in ampules containing 100 milligrams

of the drug in 20 milliliters of solvent. How many milliliters of the drug do you administer assuming the patient weighs 176 pounds?

11. The patient in problem 10 should receive an infusion of amrinone following his bolus. How many drops per minute should you administer to deliver 5 micrograms per kilogram per minute if you place 100 milligrams of amrinone in 500 milliliters of D_5W?

12. You are to administer 3 milligrams of verapamil to a patient. The drug is supplied in 2-milliliter ampules containing 5 milligrams of the drug. How many milliliters of the drug do you administer?

Answers to Practice Conversions on page 296

1. 0.75 kilogram
2. 45 milligrams
3. 650 milliliters
4. 0.1 milligram
5. 76.4 kilograms
6. 109.2 centimeters
7. 2750 milliliters
8. 20°C
9. 75 milligrams
10. 375 milliliters
11. 8.2 kilograms
12. 1000 liters
13. 113°F
14. 0.25 (¼) grain
15. 5 grains

Answers to Drug Dosage Calculations on page 297

1. 1.25 milliliters
2. 4 milliliters
3. 2 milliliters
4. 1.5 milliliters
5. 0.8 milligrams/milliliters
6. 150 drops per minute
7. 83.3 drops per minute
8. 3 milliliters
9. 200 drops per minute
10. 12 milliliters
11. 120 drops per minute
12. 1.2 milliliters

INDEX

A

$$\begin{array}{r} 31.2 \\ 25{\overline{\smash{\big)}\,17.80}} \end{array}$$